WAYS YOU CAN HELP

CREATIVE, PRACTICAL SUGGESTIONS
FOR FAMILY AND FRIENDS
OF PATIENTS AND CAREGIVERS

MARGARET COOKE
WITH ELIZABETH PUTMAN

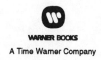

WARNER BOOKS

A Time Warner Company

Copyright ©1996 by Margaret R. Cooke
All rights reserved.

Warner Books, Inc., 1271 Avenue of the Americas, New York, NY 10020

 A Time Warner Company

Printed in the United States of America

First Printing: April 1996

10 9 8 7 6 5 4 3 2 1

Library of Congress Cataloging-in-Publication Data
Cooke, Margaret R.
    Ways you can help : creative, practical suggestions for family and
  friends of patients and caregivers / Margaret Cooke, with
  Elizabeth Putman.
      p.   cm.
   ISBN 0-446-67125-8
   1. Care of the sick—Psychological aspects. 2. Caregivers.
  3. Helping behavior.   I. Putman, Elizabeth. II. Title.
R726.5.C675 1996
362. 1—dc20   95-3524
                                                CIP

Designed by Eli Hardof
Cover design by Julia Kushnirsky

**Dedicated to
Nicholas**

Acknowledgments

Many people have contributed to this book with their experiences, good and bad. We met them in hospital waiting rooms, clinics, and support groups. Each had a special story to tell. In some cases we will never know their names as the stories grew out of casual conversations before this book was even an idea; others were related by friends and coworkers who had particular experiences they wanted to share. We offer a special thank you to everyone who helped in the creation of this book.

The following people should receive special recognition for their contributions:

Marie Kingdon for the wealth of ideas she offered and her support throughout the project.

Beth Ferguson who loaned the computer on which this book was written. It literally would not have been done without her.

Mary Elizabeth Low and Ray Joseph who provided invaluable advise and support.

Jackie and Jill Black, Maggie Miller, Sandy Svec, and Karen Wenk who provided perspective and an extensive account of their personal experiences.

And a special thank you to our editors, Anne Hamilton and Diana Baroni.

In memory of John Kingdon and John Putman.

Contents

FOREWORD: OUR STORY

The date was Thursday, June 17, 1993; it was 4:20 P.M. I had just walked into my office from a series of meetings when my secretary said that Buffy, my niece who lived in town, was on the line. Strange, I thought; she usually calls me directly on the phone at my desk, rather than bothering my secretary with a family call.

Buffy needed a favor. Would I pick up the children from her pediatrician's office and let them play at my house while she and her husband, Dan, met with the doctor?

I was out the door before I considered the obvious question "Why did the doctor want to talk with them?" I thought about nothing else as I drove across town. Buffy and the children—Jessica, seven, and Nicholas, three—were in the parking lot when I arrived. She was as serious as I'd ever seen her, and offered few details.

I learned that Dan had taken Nicholas to the doctor for his routine three-year-old well-baby exam and that the blood test results were not right. The doctor then asked to speak to both parents and suggested that someone take the children for a while. I arrived at five o'clock—dinnertime—so I decided to take the children to McDonald's, and Buffy agreed to meet us there after the meeting.

We selected one of Nicholas's favorite spots, the McDonald's that featured Oldsmobile products built in Lansing. I thought the displays and decorations would keep the children occupied if their parents' meeting ran longer than expected. We found an empty booth decorated with headlights and running boards. We ordered, ate dinner, and enjoyed the surroundings. We were in no hurry. But Buffy and Dan did not arrive. We ordered dessert; still no sign of them.

We had exhausted all the restaurant had to offer, so we went on to my house, which was nearby. We played with the toys I kept for the children's visits, then the piano, the dog; we even went for a walk. Nicholas grew tired, so we had to turn back. It was seven thirty, and still no parents. My stomach was in knots, and the novelty of visiting Aunt Margie had worn off long ago for the children.

Then the phone rang. In a very flat voice, Buffy explained that the blood test showed that Nicholas had leukemia, and they would be taking him to the hospital that evening to begin treatment. They were packing his things now; could Jessica stay with me?

Thus began our family saga.

On the day of the diagnosis, Buffy's parents were in Switzerland and Dan's mother was in California. Buffy's brother, John, and his wife, Katie, were the only other relatives in the area, and they were an hour away.

After Buffy and Dan picked up Nicholas, Jessica and I tried to make sense of what had occurred. It had all happened so suddenly. Nick had not been sick. They had just gone to the doctor for a checkup.

I knew Buffy and Dan needed someone with them at the hospital, and I thought of the rector from our church. Who better at a time like this? I realized it would be difficult to explain the situation with Jessica sitting next to me, so I called Marie, a special friend from church, and gave her a brief outline of Nick's condition. She understood immediately what was needed and made the call to the rector. He went directly to the hospital.

John and Katie arrived later that evening and took over Buffy's house, cleaning, doing the laundry, and caring for the dog.

The next morning Marie arrived at my house with a fresh fruit plate, her VHS VCR so I could rent movies for Jessica (I had a Beta), and a toy for Nicholas. Then she cleaned the kitchen so Jessica and I could write a story for Nick. My work staff arrived later with a huge plate of cold cuts, assorted breads, pickles, potato chips, and two dozen chocolate chip cookies. This plate kept the whole family in sandwiches for days!

As the word spread, friends and acquaintances called Buffy's home and mine with offers of help. It was clear that people wanted to support our family and to assist in any way they could. Some brought food or provided other assistance without being told, but most did not know specifically what to do. They wanted direction and guidance from the family, but we were too involved with our crisis to provide the needed direction.

Nick was in the hospital for over a month, and after a few days the crisis became the routine. The grandparents arrived, the church organized a committee to provide dinners, and many friends offered help in more ways than we ever dreamed possible. Yet it was also striking how many people truly wanted to help but held back through fear of intruding, overstepping, or doing the wrong thing. They wanted to know what would be useful before they did anything, for fear of making a mistake. Later we heard that some were afraid they didn't know us well enough to step in at such a personal time.

Perhaps in the days of large extended families, there was not the need for help from friends and acquaintances at times of family emergencies. In the nineties, however, families are spread all over the country, even the world. We must depend on neighbors, friends, and coworkers to fill the support gap.

One night it came to me—why not write a book about ways people *can* help when illness strikes someone close to them. We would offer simple, practical advice for reaching out to those who are ill and to their families.

I knew we had the qualifications to write this book. My father was a diabetic. I had rheumatic fever as a child and was diagnosed with multiple sclerosis in 1980. I also had major surgery a few years ago. My mother was ill for several years with heart trouble, and my grandmother and uncle both needed nursing home care. Dan's father died after a long bout with cancer. At many times in our lives we had needed the support of others, and it had been there. It seemed that this book would be a way for our family to heal from the tragedy of Nicholas's illness and give a gift to others based on our experience.

We are pleased to report that Nicholas is in remission and is getting along very well. He had several months of intensive chemotherapy, but is now in a maintenance phase of chemotherapy, which will last for two more years. He is a normal, active boy, into Power Rangers and Teenage Mutant Ninja Turtles, and he recently celebrated his fifth birthday.

Introduction

Your neighbor's child is diagnosed with a life-threatening illness. An older friend enters a nursing home. Chronic disease strikes a member of your family. A coworker has a heart attack.

What can you do to help?

Whether the person who is ill is a close friend, a relative, an acquaintance you don't know well but like a lot, or a coworker, it is natural to want to reach out, to make it better or at least to let her know you care. Yet often we are hesitant to act. We don't know what to do or are concerned we'll do the wrong thing. We don't want to intrude. We feel we might get in the way, or we assume the family has other people helping who know them better than we do. Perhaps we feel we have been out of touch too long and that it would be inappropriate to call when something bad has happened. "She wouldn't want to hear from me now."

Sound familiar? Many of us have limiting thoughts that keep us from reaching out when we are truly needed.

If you're one of those people, this book is for you. In addition to presenting numerous ways you can help, we also hope to give you the permission and confidence you need to offer that help.

What we heard again and again from both patients and their families was that any gesture is appreciated—from a greeting card, to making dinner, to some of the more creative ideas we discuss in this book. No one kept track of how long it had been since they'd heard from that friend. It truly is the thought that counts.

The other message that came through loud and clear was "Just do it!" People in crisis are not able to give direction on things that need to be done. If they are lucky, a friend or relative is able to take charge, but more often the family just muddles through as best they can.

Ways You Can Help presents concrete, practical ideas that can be used when help is needed. Many of the ideas are not new but are included as reminders and as a handy reference for things both small and large that can make a difference.

The book is divided by age—children, teenagers, and adults—and by circumstances—long-term illness, new baby, nursing homes, and the chronically and terminally ill. It will help you provide support for the family of a person who is ill and for the primary caregiver, the siblings, or the children of the patient, and offers tips on visiting. Also included is a discussion of situations when it is difficult to offer help and special situations that require innovative solutions.

It is important to realize that many of the ideas presented will apply in several different circumstances. For instance, while a child will love a life-size balloon figure, an adult might also find that same balloon a great gift.

The categories were designed to make the book easy to use and to ensure that the ideas presented are appropriate for each situation. To gain the maximum value from the book, however, we recommend that you browse through the entire contents, as you may find just the right idea for your particular circumstance where you least expect it.

In writing a book of this kind, we had to consider all situations and circumstances; therefore, we approached the topic from the assumption that the patient was alone or had no one, no spouse or other live-in helper, to perform needed tasks like errands and house-keeping. In this way we were able to provide the broadest range of ideas for ways to help.

The use of proper pronouns is a challenge to the nineties writer. In an effort to create a text that is as clear as possible, the gender pronouns "he" and "she" have been alternated by chapter. In each case the pronoun is meant to refer to both men and women. When gender-specific ideas are presented, they are labeled as such.

We have tried to keep repetition to a minimum, but in some cases it was necessary to include similar ideas in more than one chapter, because they are appropriate in several circumstances.

Many anecdotes are from our personal experience, while others are stories shared with us by people who have faced similar situations. The names that are used have been changed so as not to embarrass anyone who shared experiences with us. We have found that while each individual story is unique, the need for help is universal.

We hope you will find *Ways You Can Help* a useful tool to assist you in providing support and assistance to families and friends in need. It has been a labor of love.

Chapter One

When a Child Is Ill

Being a sick child is no fun—not for the child, not for the parents, and not for the other family and friends who try to help.

The normally active child must now stay in bed or be confined to his house. A very young child won't understand why he can't play with his friends, while an older child often feels isolated and left out.

Anyone who has attempted to keep a child entertained at home for several days or weeks knows what a true challenge is. Finding creative alternatives to keep the child from becoming bored is a full-time job. Fresh ideas, faces, and activities are essential.

Mail a Greeting

All children love to receive letters and cards. Cards require little time to send but mean so much to the child at home.

A friend of mine from work sent Nicholas several cards when he was undergoing chemotherapy. He didn't know her, but was thrilled each time her card arrived. That's the nice thing about cards; you don't have to know a child well to send one. If you learn that a friend or coworker's child is ailing, just drop a card in the mail. It's a small effort with a big reward.

Make It a Habit

If possible, send cards regularly throughout an illness. For instance, send one every Monday. Or consider sending a card every day the child is in the hospital.

I maintain a supply of cards for all occasions, so I am always prepared. I prop the cards on their sides in a shoe box so I can flip through easily to find one that is appropriate.

Do It Yourself

It isn't necessary to pay for professionally-made cards. You can create a special greeting with paper or cardboard and colored pencils or crayons, pictures cut from magazines, or other artistic materials like glue and glitter.

Cards can also be made by a school or church class, or the classmates can paint pictures with special messages. Children involved in a project for a friend learn to be thoughtful of others while enjoying a fun activity. One classroom made a life-size poster on which each child painted a picture or wrote a special message. It became a decoration for the sick child's room as well as a reminder of his friends.

Reach Out by Phone

The telephone fascinates children, especially younger children. They like to play with the phone and will be thrilled if a call is actually for them. But be prepared: With small children the call may last only twenty seconds. Children are not great conversationalists; they'll just like the idea that they received a call.

The phone is also an important way to stay in touch with an older child. You can find out how he is feeling and solicit gift ideas, while creating a break in his routine. A young girl with a broken arm was able to share by phone with her grandparents the disappointment that she had been unable to share with her parents about missing a week at camp. Once she expressed her feelings, she felt better and was then able to talk to her folks.

Encourage the child to call you as well. Phone companies offer gift certificates, which make wonderful gifts. A child of seven or eight will feel quite grown up to receive phone certificates to call a grandparent, relative, or friend long distance.

...And in Person

Visits break the monotony of a day at home or in the hospital. Even if you can only stay for a few minutes, you will be a welcome diversion for both parents and children. If you can stay a while and help either in entertaining the child or with some household task that is needed, all the better.

Keep in mind that it is the child who is sick, so give him your major attention. Take time to talk with him, play a game, or bring a special treat. Let him know he is your primary reason for being there.

When I was sick as a child, a friend of my mother's dropped by every week to see me. She always took the time to play a game with me or to read a story; then she had coffee with my mother. Her visits meant a great deal, and I still think of her fondly.

If the child is confined to his room at home or in a hospital, place a large poster board on one wall. As visitors come by, have each person sign his name and trace his hand or draw a little picture. It will be fun to see how fast the poster fills up. It also shows the child how many people had "a hand" in making him better.

It is important for even a very young child to interact with friends his own age. When the child's condition permits, arrange visits from friends and classmates. Adults make good company, but there is no substitute for peers who share common interests and experiences.

Children hate to be different, and being sick makes you different. You can't play hard like the other kids, you miss class and school activities, and you may have limits when you return to school. The ability to see friends and to share experiences on a regular basis keeps the child from becoming lonesome or feeling left out.

Visits by Tape

If personal visits are not possible, encourage friends to record their greetings on video- or audiotape. A class could have a special-credit assignment to tape a video for a sick friend. Videotaping favorite spots, hangouts, parks, games, or other special events is another way to keep the child a part of activities he can't attend in person.

One class recorded messages on an audiotape and took pictures of each member who spoke. The pictures were then mounted on a large poster board that was hung in the sick child's room. It served as a daily reminder that the child was still part of the group.

Create a Little Magic

Joy comes easily to children. Seeing a child smile when you bring a special gift or surprise will make your day.

It is often a concern that too many presents will spoil the child. Speaking as a child who spent a lot of growing-up years at home ill, I say not to worry. A package of stickers or a small toy can give a sick child hours of entertainment and will let him know he is loved. If he seems to be looking forward more to the present than to your visit, come without a gift the next time; my guess is that he will still be happy to see you.

Hire a clown, magician, or similar entertainer just for him, or hire a caricaturist to draw his picture.

Surprise him with a ride to get an ice-cream cone, see the sunset, watch a train go by, or see planes land at the airport. Any short trip will help the time pass and will create a welcome change of scenery.

Bring a musical instrument when you visit, and entertain the child and his family. A singalong is always fun, and the whole family can participate. If you have no special skills, bring a friend with a special talent to do the entertaining.

Have a life-size balloon of a favorite cartoon character delivered to the house. These balloons last weeks and provide a wonderful playmate. Nicholas received a Teenage Mutant Ninja Turtle balloon while he was in the hospital. It became his special buddy and he took it everywhere.

Dress up in a friendly costume and bring a surprise meal or treat. Children love dress-up. Bring a mask for him to wear.

Let the Imagination Work

Imagination seems to be at its peak during childhood. When the child is ill, his imagination can be used both to entertain him and to help him deal with his illness.

Writing stories is a creative way for the child to express his feelings and thoughts. Ask him to tell the story while you write it down, or make one up together. Ask him to illustrate the story as well.

Bring photos from home, and ask him to make up a story based on the scenes in the pictures.

Read a story and then ask the child to write his own story based on what you have just read, or just read him a story. Reading is something children always enjoy, and it helps them be quiet so they can rest.

Select ideas that will involve the child in the activity whenever possible. Play a game. Sing a song. Paint the child's face. Paint your face. Play charades. Work with him on a jigsaw puzzle. Color a picture together. It is important that the child be as active as his condition permits.

Tell and exchange jokes, riddles, knock-knock jokes, rhymes, and poems. Buy a joke book, or just make up jokes together, the sillier the better. Laughter truly is the best medicine.

Use arts and crafts projects to help the sick child feel a sense of accomplishment and enjoy spending time with you. Teach him what you know—knitting, needlepoint, crocheting, constructing a model, carving, calligraphy. Any special skill that you have may be of interest to the child.

I learned many of my favorite hobbies when I was home sick as a child. My grandmother taught me needlepoint, knitting, and canasta. My parents taught me bridge. I also learned the value of jigsaw puzzles at a young age.

Baking cookies is another great pastime. If you don't have time to mess with all the ingredients, buy logs of cookie dough and decorate the cookies as they come from the oven. The logs are not only a time-saver, but also allow you to bake only what is needed at any one time. Several days of fun can come from just one package.

If the child has an interest in cooking, look in the bookstores for "kids-only" cookbooks that provide simple recipes a child can make from ingredients usually found in the home. Have the child help with dinner, using some of the special recipes from his cookbook.

Make costumes or special outfits—cowboy, sailor, princess. By working with you, the child can learn the basics of sewing.

Decorate hats together. Glue beads, buttons, or fabric patches onto an old baseball cap, or use feathers and ribbon to update an old hat from the attic.

Help the child paint pictures to decorate his sickroom. These pictures can be rotated weekly or daily to provide a new look for the room.

Trace letters and stencils, or work on an art project together. Painting plaster or ceramic figurines is another way for the child's creativity to be expressed.

In many cases the hospital will allow children to paint the windows of their rooms with washable paint. You can do the same thing at home. It helps personalize his space and gives him a visible accomplishment to show off to visitors. Be sure the paint is washable!

Be Patient

One caution before we go further: Children are painfully honest. If they don't feel like doing a particular thing, they won't do it. In our house we call it "You can't make me have fun"—which means "I'm not going to enjoy myself even if you try to make me!" The last thing you want is to force the child to participate in an activity when he doesn't want to. You can offer ideas and suggest things the two of you can do together, but don't be hurt if the child is not interested. Remember: He is sick and may not feel like an activity at that particular moment. Don't be discouraged. Try, try again.

When Nicholas first came home from the hospital, a friend who is a professional clown offered to visit him on a Sunday afternoon. I thought he would be thrilled, but when she arrived he would have none of her. She offered to paint faces, and after everyone else in the family had been suitably decorated, he finally joined in. In the end he had a good time, but it was a struggle.

Emotional Outlets and Support

Children have difficulty expressing their thoughts and feelings to grown-ups, especially when they are ill. It is likely that the child is dealing with a situation he has never faced before. If he is very ill, he is certainly afraid. He may not understand what is happening to him, and not know what questions to ask to find out. One way to help the child communicate is to give him a journal to record his feelings. He can use it to write down his thoughts, what he is feeling, or just what happened during the day. This is a way for the child to collect questions that can then be asked of the doctor or a parent later.

If the child is too young to write, you may be able to help by writing in the book as he talks. You can also develop questions that he can answer, to stimulate his thinking: What do you like most about being home sick? What don't you like so much? What is your favorite toy? What would you like to do most when you get well?

Puppets are another means to help the younger child express his feelings and emotions. By talking through a puppet, a child may say things he has been keeping inside or would be afraid to say without the puppet for cover.

It is also important to be a good listener. If you can help the child talk about his feelings, you may be able to discover the things that are bothering him. The doctor should also take time to listen to the child's concerns and to answer questions fully. The imagination has a way of taking over if information is absent.

Gift Ideas

Children have short attention spans, so gifts that amuse and provide a fresh source of entertainment are best. A selection of gift ideas follows. Most are acceptable for a range of ages. If you are not sure what would be best for a particular child, ask his parents.

- ❤ Funny slippers or socks
- ❤ Pajamas or nightgown
- ❤ Fun bathrobe
- ❤ Flowers or a plant in a decorative container
- ❤ Videos—movies and games
- ❤ Cassettes or CDs of cheerful music
- ❤ Pillows
- ❤ Books
- ❤ Radio
- ❤ Walkman
- ❤ Coloring books
- ❤ Crayons, colored pencils, or markers
- ❤ Doctor kit
- ❤ Dolls
- ❤ Stuffed animals
- ❤ Puppets
- ❤ Dollhouse
- ❤ Small cars
- ❤ Games
- ❤ Playing cards
- ❤ Jigsaw puzzles
- ❤ Special food treats (make sure he is not on a restricted diet)
- ❤ Trading cards
- ❤ Bedsheets with favorite characters

- Hobby-related items
- Handheld electronic games
- Etch-a-Sketch
- Airplanes
- Scrapbook
- Stickers
- Joke books
- Jacks
- Marbles
- Play dough
- Bubbles
- Paper dolls
- Special cup and straws
- Hats—especially important if the child is undergoing chemotherapy
- Costumes

When shopping for appropriate activities, books, and games, consider those targeted to children who will be traveling. They provide activity ideas that can be done in a confined space and that usually are not strenuous. Activities books for rainy days may also have useful ideas.

If you are concerned that the child has too many toys, give him a piggy bank and add change each time you visit. Others will also contribute, and he may be able to save enough money by the time he is well to buy a special treat.

For a Long-term Illness

Most ideas in this chapter are appropriate regardless of the length of time the child will be confined at home or in the hospital. We have developed chapter 2 as a separate chapter covering long-term illness, however, because a child who is ill for months or years requires a special level of attention and innovation.

In Closing

When a child is ill it is important that he be entertained, involved, and stimulated to learn.

What Can You Do to Help?

- ✓ Stay in touch by phone, fax, mail, or in person.
- ✓ Organize others—classes, church groups, teams, and friends—to keep in contact by making cards, sending other greetings by audio- and videotape, and visiting whenever possible.
- ✓ Create surprises with gifts, activities, and short trips.
- ✓ Be patient. Understand that a sick child may not be on his best behavior.
- ✓ Develop projects and activities that use the imagination and teach new skills in an entertaining way. Do them together.
- ✓ Pay attention to the child's emotional side. Be there to listen, and offer ways he can express his feelings.

Chapter Two

When the Child Has a Long-term Illness

A young child who is seriously ill does not understand the ramifications of words like "chronic," "terminal," or "long-term." It either hurts or it doesn't; she feels good or she doesn't. Parents may face worries about their sick child's future, but she is not concerned with the long term; she only cares about how things are today.

The challenge for all who care for the child is to create an environment similar to the one she would have if she were well, with opportunities to learn, play, and grow. Allowing the sick child to be a child in an atmosphere where her kidself can grow and flourish is the most important goal.

This chapter adds to and repeats in more detail the information contained in chapter 1. Be sure to look at that chapter for other ideas for reaching out to children who are ill.

Staying in Touch

Establish a routine of sending cards, balloons, or flowers. Rotate what you send: a card one week, a balloon arrangement the next. Life-size balloons make wonderful gifts and last several weeks.

Send a card every day the child is in the hospital or at other special times, such as when she is undergoing chemotherapy. Visit regularly. Call. By whatever means you can, let the child know she is in your thoughts and part of your life.

One mother told us how her daughter brightened every time the mail carrier came into her hospital room. "He didn't have a white coat, and he was bringing something special just for her."

Arrange for the child's class to send cards. For Valentine's Day and other special holidays, many classes set up a box for each child in which the other children put cards and messages. Be sure the child who is out of school is also included. Don't assume the teacher will remember. She has a lot on her mind, so a gentle reminder may be in order. Offer to pick up the cards and deliver them at the end of the school day.

I missed Valentine's Day every year of grade school because of illness. Only one class remembered me and sent a box of Valentines— Miss Higgins's third grade. The child will never forget being remembered.

Classmates can be encouraged to reach out and include the child in many ways. They can paint pictures or make cards and posters. A class assignment might be to think of new ways they can remember the child who is sick. Not only will this thoughtfulness be appreciated by the child and her family, it will also teach the children in the class the importance of caring about others.

In one middle school, thirteen fifth-grade boys shaved their heads when their buddy lost his hair during chemotherapy. The boy was quoted in *People* magazine as saying, "What my friends did made me feel stronger. It helped me get through this. I was really amazed they would do something like this for me."

As hair loss is a usual side effect of chemotherapy, assorted baseball caps and hats make great gifts. Send one when you travel to a new state or town; buy caps of favorite sports teams; cover a cap with pins or buttons of favorite hobbies, political candidates, makes of cars, or other interest areas. Make the hats fun to receive and wear.

Pretending

Pretending is a wonderful way to create a change in the child's environment, and often it can bring out feelings she has been unable to express. Through pretending, the child can be anywhere she chooses to be, doing whatever she likes.

Create a fictional character who looks after the child or takes her on adventures. My father created Constant Habit, a bunny who watched after me when I was sick and got into terrible scrapes along the way. Daddy would tell me stories, and together we decided what Constant and his home looked like. Constant Habit was my secret buddy, and I felt safer knowing he was there.

Pretend you are attending a movie. Rent a favorite video, make popcorn, set the chairs in a line like a theater row (the bed or couch can be one of the chairs or its own row).

Around the bed, set up children's kitchen appliances or other large-size toys that will allow the child to play make-believe even if she is confined to bed. With cardboard boxes and a little paint, it is possible to construct many settings in which the child can play. Cut out large pictures of animals to make a zoo, or turn the bed into a truck with headlights and a steering wheel. The opportunities are endless.

A dollhouse is another toy that is easily enjoyed in bed. I always had my dollhouse close at hand by my bed or in my playroom, wherever I was able to play.

If the child is allowed out of bed, make a fort—a card table covered with a blanket. The child can "hide" inside and create her own space. This was one of my favorite escapes. It truly provides a feeling of privacy—a rare commodity for a sick child.

Give the child dress-up clothes, old clothes you don't wear anymore, or things from your attic. Formals, jewelry, and high heels are favorites for girls; cowboy boots and hats thrill little boys. Dress up yourself. Write your own play or situation in which you can all participate, or pretend you are on a great adventure.

Using Technology for Homemade Entertainment

In today's technological age there are many ways to use cassette tapes and videos to entertain.

Prepare your own video—especially if you live far away. Have your family record messages to the child, or select a song and sing it together. Videotape your yard, dog, or sandbox, what your children made in school, or anything else that would be of interest to the child.

Record a greeting on an audio cassette—arrange for members of a class, church school, team, or other group to record individual greetings on a tape. Take pictures of the group to hang in the child's room.

Create a video travelogue of the child's favorite spots: the zoo, the park, even an amusement park or museum. If the zoo has a new animal display or a new putt-putt golf course has recently opened, make a video so the child can keep up with what's happening in the community.

Film a school sports event, such as a soccer or Little League game in which her friends are participating. Invite a few team members to the house to talk about the game when the tape is shown.

Give the child a box camera she can use to take pictures around her house or of visitors. This idea works very well in the hospital, too. Take the film to be developed; then help the child put the pictures in a scrapbook. The quality of the pictures doesn't matter; it is the act of taking them, and then seeing them developed, that is exciting to the child.

Computers are another technological advance the child can put to good use. The child can improve her computer skills, learn new programs, or just play games with her home computer. She can write letters, keep a journal, and do her homework with this handy machine.

Creating Surprises

Surprises are an essential part of childhood and provide a special lift to any child who is homebound.

Hold a surprise party for no reason. It may be that only the immediate family attends, but with decorations and special food it will feel like a special event. To make it more fun, wear masks or costumes, or let the child dress in a special outfit.

Leave little surprises at the front door, signed "A Secret Pal" or an imaginary friend. These gifts don't have to be big—stickers, a bottle of bubbles, a small car, or any little reminder will do the trick. Similar surprises can also be sent through the mail.

Create a month of surprises, similar to an Advent calendar, in which the child opens a window, a bag, or box each day to find a special treat. Again, there is no need to be fancy; a small piece of chocolate or a plastic ring will do. The idea is to give the child the anticipation of something special each day.

Invite a firefighter, police officer, or other local hero to visit, or arrange for a tour of the firehouse if her condition permits.

Set up a special project that you can work on together every time you visit. The child will know you are coming again, and you won't have to think of new things to do.

Creating a Nature Experience Inside

Learning is an essential component of childhood and should continue even if the child is ill. Science and nature provide important educational experiences and give the child fun along the way.

For ideas of interesting science experiments that can be done at home, contact a local science museum or the child's science teacher. Books on home experiments are also available at the local library or bookstore.

Here are some ideas to get you started.

- ♥ Establish an ant colony. Kits or instructional books found in hobby shops or science-related stores will show how to set up the colony and will describe the lessons that can be learned from watching the colony perform its daily tasks.

- ♥ Install an aquarium in the sickroom. There are many books about fish, and you can select a variety that will teach as well as amuse.

- ♥ Inside, in the late winter, plant a window garden or seeds that can be transplanted to the garden in the spring. The child will enjoy watching them grow a little each day.

- ♥ Hang a bird feeder outside the sickroom window. Be sure to keep it filled and squirrel-free.

- ♥ Rent nature videos and hang posters of wildlife settings in the sickroom. A child can be transported to the Grand Canyon, an African safari, or the Swiss Alps just by watching a video.

If you are not sure of the video's content, watch it first yourself. I rented a movie about the life of an otter that I thought would be great for children, but the otter was killed rather violently near the end of the movie. I decided the story wasn't right for a child who had hours in bed to think of little else.

Decorations

Changing decorations or moving the furniture in the sickroom can create a new environment and attitude.

Posters are an inexpensive way to change the artwork in a room. Use posters of dogs or cats, seasons, or favorite sayings to change the room's atmosphere. Paintings by the child or her friends also bring inexpensive art into the child's room.

Pictures of friends, family, and pets can be used to decorate the walls and tables. Change them on a regular basis. Blow up pictures of family or of special vacation places to poster size for wall hangings.

Crepe paper, balloons, and similar party decorations can also be used to create a festive mood. This type of decoration might be most appropriate when a milestone in the illness is passed, like the end of chemo, doctor's permission to take a ride, or graduation to a walking cast.

Using Special Themes to Inform and Entertain

Create themes around poster decorations; then rent or borrow videos about the topic. For instance, select a country of the world that is of interest to the child, for example, Italy. Buy posters of major attractions like St. Paul's Basilica, the Leaning Tower of Pisa, or cities like Naples, Rome, and Milan. Rent or borrow a video about Italy, a movie that was filmed there, or a concert by a famous Italian entertainer such as Pavarotti. Fix an Italian meal and invite friends who have visited the country to talk about their experience. You can even rent a foreign-language tape or borrow one from the library.

In addition to travel, themes can be developed around:

- ❤ Sports, for example, baseball: Hang posters of stars, collect baseball cards, watch a favorite team on TV, have hot dogs for dinner.
- ❤ Hobbies, like hot air balloons: Use posters of balloons, watch a videotape of a balloon race, fix a meal of things you could take to eat on a balloon ride.
- ❤ Careers, for instance, astronaut: Hang space posters, rent movies like *The Right Stuff* or documentaries of the men landing on the moon.
- ❤ School subjects, like American history: Use posters of historic places, videos on the Revolution or the Civil War, costumes, and food eaten at various times in history. Biographies of famous people are an interesting way to learn history. Ask a librarian for biographies that would be suitable to the child's age.

Keep an encyclopedia, dictionary, and globe or atlas nearby so the child can look things up when questions arise. She may learn as much from this research as from the other materials.

Pointing toward the Future

Depending on the child's medical condition, try to do as many things as possible that she would do if she were well. Take a ride in the car, get an ice-cream cone, or go for a walk, if only for half a block. Get outside. Even if she can't be out for a long period of time, the fresh air and sunshine will be invigorating.

Bring another child to play—it will be a good learning experience for both children. The child you bring should understand the situation and should be old enough to accept that her friend may not be herself or may tire easily.

Bring a small dog or puppy to visit, if there is not one in the home. Before all the cat lovers say "Don't forget the kitties," let me explain my preference for dogs. The goal is to provide an animal who will give the child affection and attention. A very friendly cat is great, but my experience with cats suggests that some can be a bit standoffish. We want a happy pet that will play with the child and come when she calls. The last thing you need is a child sobbing because the cat is hiding under the bed and won't come out!

Make a coupon book—things that can be redeemed as the child gets better: ice-cream cone, dinner at a favorite restaurant, car ride, movie, museum, sports event, or a trip to an amusement park. Include things that will give the child something to look forward to.

Food as Fun

When there are no dietary restrictions, create special delights with food. If the child is having trouble eating or isn't hungry, you may find she has more interest if the meal is special.

Cut a sandwich to look like a smiley face or create other designs with food. Make the meal fun.

Have the child help with dinner or cook the meal herself using a kid's cookbook. She may have a better appetite if she has made the meal or has contributed to its preparation.

Order a pizza to be delivered—but tell the parents it's coming!

Bake a giant cookie, or help the child bake cookies.

Bake cupcakes or cookies, and let the child decorate them. In addition to colored frosting, use M & Ms, sprinkles, colored sugars, and so on.

Coloring eggs is not just for Easter.

Fix a favorite meal or dessert. Don't be discouraged, however, if the child doesn't eat much. Sometimes what may sound good doesn't taste as great when it is actually served. It can be frustrating to make a meal and then have the child not eat it. Nicholas came for lunch while he was in the middle of chemotherapy. I fixed all his favorite foods: spaghetti, egg salad sandwiches, and ice cream. After a bite of each he was done, so you know what I had as leftovers for the next several days. The idea of the party was to get him out of his house for a special treat. That objective was met, and it was a great day. It didn't matter that he wasn't hungry.

Bring in a favorite fast-food meal. One thing homebound children don't get as often as other kids is fast food, and they love it.

Have a picnic on the living-room floor. Spread out a tablecloth, and eat food that would normally be served at a picnic. Make flies out of paper to create a more realistic scene. Cut black construction paper in the shape of a fly (body and wings are fine), or use white paper and color it black. Then use tape to stick the flies around the room, or lay them on the blanket. You can also use thread or string to hang a few from a lamp.

Create an adventure, such as a scavenger hunt with items that can be found in the house. A treasure hunt with special food and gifts at the end is also a fun activity for a small group.

Sharing Thoughts and Feelings

Give the child a journal she can use to write down her feelings and experiences: things she liked about being home and things she didn't like; plans for when she is well. Writing and thinking about her experience may help her understand her feelings and cope better. You can write it for her if she is too young or ill to write, but the thoughts must be hers.

The child can also use the journal to make lists and to develop ideas of things she would like to learn, places she would like to visit, or things to see in her own community.

Make a scrapbook of cards she has received.

Add the child to a prayer list—at her church and/or your own.

Especially for Girls

Have a makeup party for the sick child, alone or with a friend. Let her use play makeup and lipsticks, put rollers in her hair, and let her fix up like the grown-ups. The girls might also enjoy dressing for dinner in old formals.

Manicure her nails or create a new hairstyle.

Hold a doll wedding. Have the child invite a few friends, and then create a wedding ceremony using a bride doll or bride costume for her regular doll. Make a wedding cake to serve after the wedding ceremony.

Especially for Boys

Turn the sickroom into a pirate's cave or fort with colored paper, stones, and twigs from the yard. It doesn't have to be perfect. Imagination will do most of the work.

In the Hospital

These ideas bear repeating for a child who is confined in a hospital.

- ♥ Place a large poster board in the child's hospital room—have all visitors and medical personnel sign it, or trace a handprint and sign.
- ♥ Bring pictures of family, friends, and pets to decorate the sickroom.
- ♥ Bring favorite toys and other familiar things from home.
- ♥ Help the child paint the sickroom walls or windows with washable paint, if the hospital permits.
- ♥ Create a goody bag with special treats: stickers, balloons,

matchbox cars, audio cassettes, crayons or markers, candy, lollipops. Include things that can be done in bed or in the limited space of a hospital room.

❤ Send cards, flowers, and balloons. Visit if possible.

❤ Stay with the child so the parents can take a break in the cafeteria or can go home for a while.

In Closing

When a child is ill for an extended period of time, adults are challenged to keep her life as normal as possible and to let her experience as much of life as her condition permits.

What Can You Do to Help?

✓ Remember the child with periodic gifts, cards, and calls.

✓ Use her imagination to create new environments, games, and special events.

✓ Teach about geography, science, and space, using room decorations, videos, books, and even menus.

✓ Create hours of fascinating play using video, audio, and computer technology.

✓ Stimulate the child's appetite with interesting meals and food-related activities.

✓ Provide opportunities for the child to express fears and concerns about her illness. Be a good listener.

✓ Encourage friends to visit when the child's condition permits.

Chapter Three

When the Child
Is a Teenager

Few of us would choose to relive our teenage years. It is a time of pushing our boundaries and making a claim for precious independence. We prefer to conform to the standards of our peers, yet we still must follow the rules our parents establish. We are weight conscious, body conscious, clothes conscious, face conscious; you name it, we're conscious of it.

When an illness or injury strikes, the teen must deal with the problems related to his condition, while trying to be a "regular guy." It can be rough.

As you look for ways to help a teen, ideas in both the chapters on adults and children are appropriate. Yet it is precisely because the teen has one foot in each world that we believe he deserves special attention.

Keeping the Bonds Strong

The goal in any illness situation is to create as normal a life as possible, but this priority takes on special significance when the patient is a teenager. So much of his life is wrapped up in friends that every effort must be made to keep those ties strong.

Encourage friends to visit. Transportation may be an issue if the friends are not of driving age. By offering to provide the transportation, you can guarantee that the visits occur, and you can keep the number of friends manageable. It is best to have friends visit a few at a time, rather than have them all come at once and tire the patient.

- ❤ Set a time when you will bring a van or car with classmates for a pizza party. Pick up the pizza and soda pop on the way.
- ❤ Organize times when classmates will study with the teen and bring him up to date on homework and school assignments.
- ❤ Invite a favorite teacher for dinner or to join classmates who are visiting.
- ❤ If the class is studying a special topic—for instance, a period of history—encourage the patient to keep up with the homework, and then invite classmates in to discuss the major themes that emerged in class discussions. This way, the teen will feel a part of the lesson and will gain valuable insights the others learned from class participation.
- ❤ Invite friends to watch favorite television programs, movies, concert videos, or sports. It's much more fun to watch a football game with friends. Buy popcorn from the local theater; it always seems to taste better.
- ❤ Set up a jigsaw puzzle, board game, or similar activity friends can do when they visit. The more activity options available, the more likely the visit will be a success.
- ❤ Look for ways friends can share the teen's experience. Let them use the crutches, wheelchair, or eye patch.

Several teens I know joined together to have a wheelchair race when a buddy was hit by a car and lost the use of his legs. The teens who participated said they learned a lot about the challenges their friend faced, but also saw that he could lead an active life even if he didn't regain the use of his legs.

Communicating by Phone

What is a teenager without a phone? The need for phone communication becomes critical when a teen is out of daily contact with friends at school. One way classmates can help is to call regularly or to organize themselves so that at least one person calls every day to bring the teen up to date on school gossip and activities. This regular communication will help relieve any isolation the ill teen may feel and will give his classmates a way to help their friend by doing what they enjoy anyway.

Illness and hospitals are difficult for many teenagers. The ill teen may be the first person in a hospital or with a serious illness that his friends have known. If a friend hesitates to visit because of fear or discomfort, the telephone may be a good solution. He can stay in touch and maintain an important friendship. It may be that once the friend is in the habit of talking by phone, he may feel more comfortable about visiting in person.

Involving the School

Many activities can involve a whole class, team, or club and can give them an opportunity to reach out to an ill friend. School sports events, plays, parties, assemblies, or other events are all good candidates for videotaping. If a video camera is not readily available to you, chances are some parent will be taping the event and will be happy to loan the tape or to make a duplicate. Have some of the teens who participated in the activity visit with the videotape and give the patient the inside story.

Have the group make a video. The teacher can use the project as an educational opportunity for the class. The class can write a script and act parts or film locations that are special to the teen.

Have computer students make a large banner that can be hung in the lunchroom to be signed by all the students, then delivered to the sick teen. The banner can also be sent to each class the teen would normally attend, along with his homework assignment sheet, and classmates in each room can sign the banner or write a personal note.

If there is a special gift the teen would like, organize a class, club, or team to give it from the group. They can organize a car wash, bake sale, or raffle to raise the money that is needed to buy a special gift, such as a VCR or CD player.

Janet's classmates bought her a cassette recorder and tapes for her stay in the hospital. They also made a tape of themselves talking to her. When the hospital noise got annoying, or if she wanted to sleep, Janet would put on the headphones and tune everything else out. Make a group greeting card signed by all the participants. This and the audiotape are particularly useful if the teen can't have company.

A school counselor I spoke with stressed the importance of keeping the teen's teachers informed of his condition, prognosis, and any special things his classmates can do to be helpful. Teachers want to work with the family to assist the teen and can do a much better job if they are aware of the situation on a regular basis.

A Time to Learn

Learning a new skill may be a positive outcome of an illness. Musical instruments, woodworking, and needle crafts are all new things a teen could learn, if he is interested. If you have any of these skills, offer to teach them to the teen, or find out what he would like to learn and find an instructor. Offer to pay for the first month's lessons; after that he can pick up the cost if he wishes to continue. That strategy allows him to try a new skill but not feel pressured to stay with it, if it turns out not to be something he likes.

If the teen is already studying an instrument, arrange for his music teacher to come to the home so he can keep up with lessons. If his music lessons come through school, and if the teacher is unable to make home visits, hire a tutor for the time the teen will be out of school.

Hire a tutor for a new subject or to help with regular studies. It is easy to fall behind when you miss classroom work, and anything that can be done to fill the gap is valuable. Better yet, be the tutor yourself, if you are current on the subject.

Design a project you and the teen can complete together. Construct a model, design a replica of a famous building, or sew a quilt. Working on a project will give you an opportunity to share time together and will provide a positive memento of his illness. It is an important lesson that we can still be productive people even if we are ill.

Rent videos on areas of interest to the teen; both documentaries and other educational programs are available on tape. The library can suggest both books and videos that are entertaining and informative on any of the teen's favorite subjects.

Larry learned French while recovering from an injury that caused a temporary loss of sight. He used the foreign language tapes as a way of entertaining himself and helping the hours pass. His parents invited friends who spoke French to visit when Larry had enough of a foundation to communicate. It was great practice. He said that learning a language kept him from being too frightened by the changes in his life.

Your state or community may have a special library or services for persons who are blind or handicapped. They will likely provide tapes for both adults and children at no cost. Check with your local library for the services available in your area.

Emotional Support

Often as young people pass through their teen years they have trouble communicating with their family. They hold back feelings and do not believe older people can understand their situation. If this is true of the teen who is ill, a journal may be a positive solution. He can write down his thoughts and feelings about his illness and convalescent period without having to share them with anyone else, unless he chooses. If he does have trouble communicating, this record of his experience will help release feelings that are locked inside.

Audiotapes are another way he can express himself. He may even use them as audio letters to family and friends, to say things he might have difficulty expressing in person.

If you find the teen feels like talking, listen. Do not judge or provide suggestions unless they are requested. Let the teen know that his feelings are valid and important.

Friends are an important emotional outlet. Encourage visits by close friends, and give the teens the space they need to communicate. If adults are always hovering around or appear to be trying to listen in, the teens will feel they can't talk honestly to each other, and emotions will stay bottled up. When a teen is sick at home, he must feel he has some personal space just as he would have if he were able to leave the house. It is a fine balance, but an important one, to keep the communication lines open.

In the Hospital

Call before you visit a teen in the hospital. He is likely to be very embarrassed if you show up when he looks his worst.

Bodily functions can be a source of discomfort to a teen anytime, but since they are the primary focus of a hospital stay, the teen may face many situations that rob him of his dignity. The best he can hope is that they won't occur in front of friends. If you are visiting when the hospital staff comes in to care for the patient, excuse yourself until they are finished.

The worst thing one young woman remembers about her stay in the hospital was a time friends were visiting and she had to use the bathroom. She was too embarrassed to ask the friends to leave, so she just held it in. It may be appropriate for parents to set up nonverbal communication signals with their hospitalized teen, so he can indicate when he needs to have company step out of the room for a few minutes.

Young friends may not know how to tell when the patient is tired, so here is another time when nonverbal communication might be helpful. It may be easier for a parent to suggest that friends let the teen rest than for the teen to risk unpopularity or embarrassment by suggesting it himself.

In many hospitals teenagers are assigned to the pediatrics floor, which can hurt their self-image. If the teenager can be involved in activities on the floor as a mentor or counselor to the younger patients, he may feel better about his room location.

Encourage the teen to play with a younger child or to teach a special skill to the younger children in the playroom. He could even serve as a playroom supervisor for a brief period. By serving as a role model for a younger child, the teen will learn to look beyond himself, and the time will feel more productive. The hospital staff could be encouraged to invite the teen to help in the playroom. He may feel he is making a more valuable contribution if he is asked to help.

When Sam was treated for a thyroid condition, the head nurse asked him to assist the aides who visited smaller children with toys and games. Sam discovered such a gift for working with children that he is now studying to be a teacher.

There may be other activities in the hospital in which the teen can participate. Talk with the staff and see what suggestions they might offer, then present the teen with some ideas, but don't push it. It won't seem like fun if he hasn't been part of the decision.

Gift Ideas

Another characteristic of the teenage years is the desire to keep up with the latest trends. Be sure your gift is the latest fad or fashion. CDs and videos should be the most recent releases. If you are not sure what to choose, ask a salesclerk to steer you to the popular releases.

Gift certificates are another option. You can be most helpful by offering to redeem the certificate for the video, CD, or cassette of his choice. This way he gets the gift to enjoy during his recovery, and you are sure the gift is exactly what he wants.

- Videos—music, movies, or games
- Videos of favorite entertainers or comedians
- Handheld computer games
- Board games—be sure to stay and play
- Comfortable clothes in the latest style
- Music—latest CDs, music videos, cassettes
- Funny books or magazines
- Fashion magazines
- Magazines or books about favorite sports or entertainment stars
- *People* magazine or similar publications

- ❤ A big balloon character, but make sure it's appropriate for a teen. Mickey Mouse won't make it!
- ❤ Makeup kit
- ❤ Gift certificates for manicures, hair styling, makeover, color analysis
- ❤ Computer games
- ❤ Jewelry
- ❤ Hair scrunchies
- ❤ Radio
- ❤ Walkman

In Closing

Illness further complicates a teen's already complex life. It makes everything harder.

What Can You Do to Help?

- ✓ Encourage peer communication in person and by phone. Create opportunities for friends to stay a part of the teen patient's life on a consistent basis.
- ✓ Keep the teen involved in school activities by videotaping special events and inviting friends to narrate the videos. Invite friends to talk about classroom discussions and ask a favorite teacher to visit.
- ✓ Make the sick time productive with special projects, help with homework, and opportunities to learn new subjects. Provide

lessons on musical instruments, or in needlework or other crafts. Borrow educational videos and books on favorite subjects from the library.

✓ Give the teen space to be himself and the privacy to interact with friends as he would if he were away from home.

Chapter Four

The Adult Who Is Ill

When an adult becomes ill, has an accident, or needs surgery, every phase of life is affected. Sick adults must figure out how to handle family and job responsibilities, routine maintenance, bills, the yard, the dog, laundry, groceries, and whatever else may need attention.

If the condition is sudden, such as a broken leg, there can be no preparation. Life begins anew at that moment. Even small tasks like picking up dry cleaning and watering plants have to be figured out.

When the condition comes on slowly, as a disease usually does, adults may feel themselves slowing down and may defer many daily responsibilities. When I first became ill with multiple sclerosis I was so tired that putting things away or even fixing a meal felt like more than I could do. Even now, when I go through a low-energy period, my house becomes cluttered and I eat a lot of crackers.

When it is planned, surgery allows some lead time to prepare, but it carries its own set of worries. Unless the outcome is virtually certain, and few are, we must prepare for our recovery with a series of unknown variables that will determine how much help we need. How long will we stay in the hospital? Will there be a lot of pain? Will we be able to get around afterward? Is it all right if we stay home alone, or will someone have to be with us all the time? These are the kinds of questions we have to plan around, and while our doctors can give us some direction, each case presents its own special challenges.

Regardless of the type of illness situation the patient faces, or how it was caused, there will be any number of ways you can help.

Organizing for Surgery

Once a patient has agreed to surgery, she begins a race to accomplish all that must be done before she is laid up. She will likely want to put her affairs in order: update records and legal papers, pay bills, straighten the house, organize closets, and arrange personal mementos. By offering to help with these tasks, you can have a great afternoon and learn more about your friend. You will also share a few laughs or tears along the way.

If the patient is apprehensive about her surgery, your presence may give her an opportunity to express her fears. Be prepared to be a listening ear, and encourage her to share her feelings openly. If she has a chance to say what she is feeling out loud, she may realize things aren't so bad. It will be an important way you can help.

Food becomes a huge issue when you are not able to cook for yourself, or don't feel like it. In preparation for recovery, some people choose to make and freeze their favorite meals ahead. It can be lonesome and a little sad to do this kind of preparation alone, so offer to help with the grocery shopping and cooking.

If the patient is too ill or is not interested in preparing meals ahead, friends may help by preparing the dishes and freezing them at the patient's home for later use.

Care of children or pets is another priority, especially if spouses, grandparents, or other relatives are not readily available to help. If care of dependents is needed, you can offer to provide the care yourself or help the patient think through her options. Just talking a situation out with a friend is often the clearest way to develop viable alternatives.

If at all possible, someone should be with the patient both before and after surgery. It can be frightening to await a surgical procedure by yourself. The imagination can take over and raise issues in the mind that are not accurate or realistic. If you can be with the patient during this time, offer to do so. She will appreciate your asking, even if other plans have been made.

Supporting the Patient in the Hospital

Flowers and plants are sent to friends in the hospital because without some personal touches a hospital room can be a very lonely, sterile place. With the addition of live floral arrangements and similar decorations, the room takes on a personality that makes it more livable. Such gifts also remind the patient that people on the outside love and care for her—a subtle get-well message.

Choosing between flowers and plants is a matter of personal taste, but the patient's preference, if known, should be the deciding factor. I love plants and feel they provide a lasting gift that can be enjoyed for years. In fact almost all the plants in my home came from times I was in the hospital, including one that has been with me since 1966! Other people believe that flowers make a better gift specifically because you don't have to take them home. Either way, your friend will appreciate the gift and the warmth it brings to the room.

One way to avoid the plant vs. flowers decision is to send balloons. Today balloon shops can make very sophisticated bouquets that last longer than flowers and require no care. Some balloon arrangements can also be a bit silly—a valued property when one is confined to a hospital bed. They always bring a smile.

Balloons also are excellent for cancer patients who may not be able to receive fresh plants or flowers.

Gift baskets are another excellent way to remember a friend. Many places will make them up and deliver them for you, and you can be quite innovative in the products you select. Consider filling the baskets with gifts made in your state, snacks and other finger food, or bath products and personal care items.

Any gift you choose tells the patient you are thinking of her even when you are not there in person. Cards serve the same purpose. It doesn't take a lot of time to write a short note or send a card, but the patient will have many hours of pleasure from the effort.

Personal visits and calls are also critical, and not just for friendship; they go a long way to speeding recovery. We always seem to feel better when we have people looking after us and caring that we get better.

Visits should be arranged at a good time for the patient. Call ahead to be sure your friend feels up to company. In this way she will be able to clean up before you come, and perhaps she can nap so she is fresh for your visit. For a full discussion of visiting, see chapter 9.

Help the patient make a list of flowers and cards she has received. Make this list your project, and update it each time you visit the patient, at the hospital or at home. Your list will be an important record when she gets ready to write thank-you notes.

Arranging for visits by others is another service you can provide for the patient. Offer to drive a mutual friend or relative who would be unable to come without transportation, or to baby-sit with a friend's children so she can visit.

Later in the chapter is a list of gifts that are appropriate for adults. In the case of a hospital visit, however, we thought Peggy's advice was particularly useful. She recommends practical items that will make the patient's hospital stay more comfortable: Bring a pillow from home and a radio or cassette recorder, with tapes and earphones, if possible. She can use them to drown out hospital noises or when she just needs to get away mentally. Bath towels or, better yet, bath sheets are another necessity, as hospital towels leave a lot to be desired in absorbency and softness. Toilet paper with aloe or extra softness is a gift that will be treasured, especially if the patient will be in the hospital any length of time.

Recovering at Home

Hospital stays are much briefer today than in years past. Patients do the majority of their recovering at home, so continuing contact after the patient leaves the hospital is vital.

The one advantage hospitals provided was human contact. At home many patients are alone all or part of the day, with visits from family and friends their only diversion. It is not the length of time you stay but rather the fact of your visit that matters.

During your visit, look for ways to entertain the patient or to start her on a project, in addition to sharing gossip and news from the outside.

- ❤ Play a card or board game. Checkers is fun and not too demanding. Chess is also a great game, if she has the energy for it.
- ❤ Help with a puzzle. Jigsaw or crossword puzzles go faster when shared.
- ❤ Read part of a book or short story. The patient may be too fatigued to read by herself; even the act of sitting and holding a book may be too much. Even adults enjoy being read to. Listen to a book on tape together.
- ❤ Write a letter or thank-you note she dictates. Offer to stamp and mail the letter as well.
- ❤ Schedule your visit to watch a concert or sporting event you both enjoy, or rent a favorite movie video and watch it together.
- ❤ Bring a dog or puppy (potty trained) to visit.

Videos and books make the time pass more quickly and often provide an opportunity to learn about a topic of interest during recovery. You can provide a genuine service by regularly bringing videos or library books to the patient. Establish a schedule of days when you will pick up these items; then she can request her favorites.

Bring current newspapers and magazines when you visit. They will provide something for the patient to do after you leave.

If there is time, help with a household chore while you are visiting. Chances are that there will be things that need to be done if the person has been laid up for any amount of time. When I took lunch to a sick friend, I noticed that her dishwasher was full of clean dishes, so I emptied it and put the dishes away.

Once at home, the patient may need rides to doctors' appointments or other commitments. If transportation will be an ongoing need, set up a schedule with friends to share the responsibility, and assure your friend that she will get where she needs to go when she needs to be there.

The Need to Eat

"Eat well-balanced meals to get your strength back," we are often told when recovering from an illness. That admonition is easier said than followed. One reason people don't eat well when they are ill is that they don't have the energy to fix a full meal. Crackers, cookies, or junk food are often substituted to address the hunger rather than the need for nutrition.

You can provide a service to a sick friend by bringing meals or by joining with others to create a regular schedule for meals to be prepared and delivered. A club, church group, or similar group of friends can organize to bring meals every night, allowing the patient to have variety in her menu without an undue hardship on any one person.

Create a special event with your meal. Have an indoor picnic with fruit, veggies, sandwiches, wine or other beverage carried in a picnic basket. You can even spread a tablecloth or sheet on the floor and pretend it's a real picnic, if the patient is able to get down that far.

Bringing in a meal is also a good reason for a short visit and an opportunity to see how things are going in the household. We have a friend who always brings homemade soup when a person is ill. She uses the occasion of dropping off the soup to see how the patient is getting along and to determine if other help is needed. If the patient appears lonely, she will stay for a while; if the patient appears tired, our friend excuses herself, saying she was just dropping off the soup, and quickly leaves.

It isn't necessary to prepare the meal yourself. As a very thoughtful friend says, "You don't have to make great brownies; just know who does!" A meal brought in from a favorite restaurant can be a wonderful surprise and an alternative for those too busy to prepare a meal from scratch.

It may be appropriate to share the meal with the patient or to sit with her while she eats. Here again you need to evaluate the situation and decide what would mean the most to her. If you bring in a meal to share, bring along some extra, and leave it in the refrigerator to be reheated later.

Life Goes On

Sick or well, the patient's life goes on. Everyday tasks must be accomplished in and around the home.

When Oscar went to the hospital suddenly, none of his spring yard work had been done. Joe, his neighbor, stepped in to clean up the yard and to plant annual flowers as Oscar did each year.

When he came home from the hospital, Oscar was thrilled to see his beautiful yard all ready for spring.

Think of the things that need doing at your house. Chances are the patient will have the same jobs to be done.

- ❤ Tidy the kitchen; wash dishes or put them in the dishwasher. Run the dishwasher if there is a full load. Unload the dishwasher and put the dishes away.
- ❤ Mow the lawn.
- ❤ Weed the garden.
- ❤ Take the dog for a walk.
- ❤ Bundle the newspapers for recycling.
- ❤ Take soda cans back to the store.
- ❤ Drop off or pick up laundry/dry cleaning; do a load of laundry.
- ❤ Take small appliances to be fixed.
- ❤ Pick up groceries and put them away.
- ❤ Pick up the house; vacuum, dust.
- ❤ Make sure there is extra toilet paper in the bathrooms.
- ❤ Take the car for an oil change; gas it up.
- ❤ Polish the silver.

You get the idea.

When you offer to help with a task, see it all the way to its final conclusion. When Sara broke her leg, a friend offered to pick up a bag of kitty litter at the store. When the friend dropped the bag off, she left it in the middle of the kitchen. Sara, who was on crutches, couldn't get around it and couldn't move it—an example of a good deed gone bad. If you aren't sure where to put things, ask.

To Help a Coworker

A person's work life can be severely altered when she becomes ill. When work piles up, coworkers who step in to fill the gaps sometimes screw things up. Sometimes the substitute does such a good job that the boss will decide she should do the job permanently.

Laws now protect a worker from being fired when she becomes ill, which was a very real possibility not so many years ago. In those times, workers often returned to work too soon in order to protect their jobs, or they were afraid to see a doctor for fear of losing time. It still happens that a worker is reassigned after an illness or finds that her duties have been moved around in her absence. Job security fears are real and need to be understood in the context of helping a coworker who is ill.

One way to alleviate undue worry is to stay in contact. It may not be reasonable for the patient to continue making day-to-day decisions, but if she knows the major issues the office has been handling, she will feel more confident when she returns. In addition she may have valuable insights that can help others do her job better.

When her condition permits, drop off mail or periodicals that she may enjoy reading while she is away. It may be a good time to catch up on articles there wasn't time to read at the office.

If the patient doesn't work in an office or have the kind of job in which updates are appropriate, coworkers can still call or visit to let the patient know she is not forgotten.

Help the patient stay a part of the team. Organize a small group of coworkers to stop by periodically for lunch or after work. Send group cards, flowers, or similar gifts. Call now and then with the office gossip.

The View from Crutches

A broken leg causes any number of inconveniences, most of which you wouldn't think about unless it happened to you. While many of the ideas below are the same as those mentioned throughout this chapter, there are a few with a slightly different slant for patients with crutches.

- Bring assorted microwave meals that the patient can heat in a few minutes. Standing on crutches for any length of time is difficult.

- Bring soda and other drinks in bottles rather than cans, so the patient can screw the top back on and move with it. Individual-sized bottles are more convenient and lighter to carry than the family size.

- Provide ziplock bags or small bags with handles to carry items in. This system works particularly well for carrying

ice and soda pop to a glass. For hot drinks, covered cups are
the answer, as again the patient can carry them while using
crutches and not cause a spill.

- Offer to water plants. It is difficult to carry a water jug while
  using crutches.
- Shovel the snow on the sidewalks and driveway. Be sure to salt
  the icy spots.

The patient will likely need transportation to appointments and
to work once restrictions are lifted. When Julia injured her leg,
coworkers assigned themselves different days to pick her up for work
in the morning and to bring her home at night. Julia didn't have to
worry about adequate transportation or take on the burden of having
to arrange every day herself.

. . . Or a Sling

We could probably have a debate on which is harder—a broken leg
or a broken arm. Needless to say, each provides its own challenges.

If an arm is broken or injured, accommodations must be made for
lifting, toting, dressing, and writing. It can be a struggle getting
clothes on and off or pouring a drink of water.

If a friend has an injured arm:

- Place food in individual containers so no pouring or measuring
  is needed. Buy beverages in individual serving containers.
- Transfer food items in cans and jars to containers that are

easily opened. Many of the plastic containers sold for leftovers are perfect.

- Loan a microwave oven if the patient doesn't have one. Microwave cooking will be much easier than trying to keep several pots going on the stove, or opening the oven door.
- Write letters the patient dictates or provide a cassette recorder and blank tapes that she can use for audio letters.
- Supply a small table, or cart with wheels, that the patient can use to transport several items from one room to the next.
- Have the pharmacist place medications in packages that do not have childproof caps.

As the Patient Improves

One of the things that surprised me was how long it took to get my strength back. If the patient has been through a particularly difficult time, it may take months before she is back to full energy, and in the interim she will appreciate opportunities to get out of the house or to have visitors.

- Take her for a ride. Just leaving the house and having a change of scenery can greatly improve her morale.
- Give a gift certificate for a manicure, pedicure, facial, or massage, and provide transportation to the appointment.
- Schedule a hairstyling or an appointment with the barber.
- Organize a bridge, poker, or monopoly game with a few

friends. Hearts is a favorite game in our family and is not hard to play even if the patient is having trouble concentrating.

💜 Create an early evening drop-in time when friends or coworkers can stop by on their way home from work. As a friend you can organize the gathering and serve as the host, so the patient doesn't feel the need to look after the guests.

Using a wheelchair, the patient may be able to visit the zoo, a garden, a park, or a movie. Often public places will have wheelchairs available, or a local hospital supply store may rent them for a nominal fee.

Gift Ideas

In addition to flowers, plants, and balloons there are many other thoughtful gifts for the adult who is ill. These include:

💜 Jigsaw puzzles, crossword puzzles
💜 Videos—new releases or a favorite classic
💜 Games of all kinds—board, computer, or video games—are all fun, and some computer and video games can be played by one person. Computer solitaire can become pleasantly addicting.
💜 Books and magazines: With reading or viewing materials, be sure the topic is of interest to the patient. What appeals to you may not to her.
💜 Telephone gift certificates

- Books on tape
- Lap desk
- Housecoat or bathrobe: Comfortable outfits that look like clothes are most appreciated.
- Nightgown, nightshirt, or pajamas: Check ahead to see which the person prefers.
- Slippers
- Pretty sheets
- Bed jacket
- Reading pillow
- Carafe with matching water glass
- A long phone cord

Marie sends each friend in the hospital a basket of small presents, one for each day she will be in the hospital. The gifts are thoughtful rather than expensive, but give the patient something to look forward to each day. Some things she includes are a small brush, hand lotion, deck of cards, magazine, or a small book of poetry. Product samples from cosmetic lines can be cute and useful gifts for a get-well basket.

Jigsaw puzzles are great gifts for a person with limited mobility but an active mind. When I was first diagnosed with MS my energy was limited, and puzzles allowed me to work at my own speed and to stop when I was tired. They challenged my mind without putting stress on my body and provided a sense of accomplishment that was important to a person who was used to being in control of her life. I give puzzles now as gifts to friends who will be laid up for a time. By the way, the five hundred-piece variety is best for a person who is in the early stages of recovery, as anything larger can be too complicated and can become discouraging. Buy puzzles that are not too challenging—you are providing a positive activity that should be easily accomplished with modest effort. I know of one man who was given a thousand-piece all-red puzzle as a gift after surgery. He never felt up to working on it, even after he was well.

In Closing

All phases of an adult's life are affected when illness strikes. The patient must deal with her illness and keep the other areas of her life moving as well.

What Can You Do to Help?

✓ Help the patient prepare for surgery by getting organized at home and by preparing meals and care alternatives for her recovery.

✓ Send cards and gifts to the hospital to personalize the room, and let the patient know she is remembered. Visit during hospital stays and while the patient is recovering at home.

✓ Bring in meals, and organize others to do the same. Provide a schedule that will let the patient know who will be bringing meals each day.

- ✓ Help with household tasks that may pile up while the patient is ill or that may have been neglected when the illness began.
- ✓ Stay in contact with a coworker who is ill, and keep her a part of the job scene through phone calls, visits, and sharing information about work.
- ✓ Provide necessary adaptive devices so a patient with an injured arm or leg can maintain a level of independence.
- ✓ As the patient improves, find ways to get her out of the house, or create a small social activity at home where she can see friends.

Chapter Five

The New Baby

A new baby presents many of the same challenges that come with an illness or operation. Usually the mother is hospitalized, and arrangements must be made for the household to function both in her absence and when she returns home with the infant. Many of the helping ideas contained in chapters 4 and 8 are appropriate in this situation, but moms I talked to also had specific ideas for things that are helpful in the last few months of pregnancy and when the new baby arrives.

The amount of help new parents receive seems to diminish after the first child. For first babies, grandparents, relatives, and friends rally around, perhaps assuming that the new parents can't handle the job. After that, they're on their own. Grandparents schedule trips, friends have other worries, and the parents are left to care for the children they already have as well as a new baby.

Whether the baby is the first or the tenth, the parents need support and help in the weeks before and after the birth. The same is true if the child is adopted. The new arrival requires adjustments in every aspect of family life. These adjustments are usually happy, but stressful nonetheless, as the family learns to adapt and change.

Preparing for the New Arrival

In the last few weeks of pregnancy, the mother-to-be may experience greater fatigue than usual and may find that her size makes it difficult to keep up with regular household duties. Yet it is important that her house be as organized as possible before she delivers, as she will need to focus her full attention on the baby when they come home from the hospital.

Helping with housework, organizing cupboards, cooking and freezing meals, putting final touches on the nursery, and packing for the trip to the hospital are useful activities that can make a fun afternoon of sharing with the mother-to-be. Catching up on the laundry is another vital job.

One mom said she appreciated company when her special cravings hit. Having her husband or a friend along made it more of an outing.

Often the mother's size or the position of the baby in the days before delivery can make driving a car difficult. Driving the mom to appointments and errands can be an important service.

Cards, visits, and calls are also appreciated if the mom is laid up for any amount of time before she delivers. People who stop by and offer to help with household tasks are lifesavers, especially if the mother-to-be is spending her days looking at things around the house that need to be done, but that she can't do herself.

At the Hospital

Babies do not arrive according to any prearranged timetable; they set their own schedule. If you are a neighbor or live close by, offer to be on call to care for children and pets when labor starts. The parents should give you a key to the house so you can come right in when called. Be prepared: The call will likely arrive in the middle of the night!

Visiting the hospital to see the new mother is best left until the day after the baby is born, unless you are a close relative or friend or the parents have specifically invited you to come. On the first day the mother will be tired, and the parents will be getting acquainted with their new child. One husband's secretary arrived at the hospital to visit two hours after the baby was born. The wife, who barely knew the woman, had just been moved to her hospital room from the delivery room. It was a most uncomfortable situation for the parents.

Hospital stays are so short these days that it may be best not to visit until mother and baby come home. The atmosphere will be more relaxed, and the mother will appreciate the company. In either case, call ahead. The mom can tell you a convenient time for a visit based on the baby's schedule, or lack of one.

Many hospitals plan a special dinner for the new parents before the mother and baby leave. If a program like this is not available at the hospital, offer to bring in a special meal for the parents on the last night. You can order take-out from a favorite restaurant or cook the meal yourself. Include candles, silverware, and champagne or sparkling juice to make the evening a festive celebration.

Shop for groceries before the new family comes home, so essentials are fresh and in place. What a relief! Do the laundry if it was not done before the trip to the hospital; it surely won't be done in the first days the baby is home.

The First Week Home

The first week at home is a major adjustment for the parents and any other children. The baby will likely not have a schedule, or may sleep all day and be awake all night. Babies can be fussy for long periods, finding little comfort in adult attempts to divert their attention.

One late-in-life dad, who had held responsible jobs and was used to control, was shocked when the new baby arrived and he had absolutely no way to make her conform to his wishes. She slept when he didn't want her to, was awake when he wanted to sleep, and generally acted like a baby. It took several weeks before he figured out he had met his match.

Most moms I know told me how helpful it was to have a supportive grandparent or aunt stay those first few days to help the parents and take a turn with walking-the-floor duties. This assistance is usually offered for the first baby, but often not for the second or third, when parents may need the help even more. If you are in a position to offer this kind of support, do it. Even if other plans have been made, it's nice to know who will be available if a backup is needed.

You don't have to sleep over to be helpful. The mom is often alone during the day and would appreciate help at that time. Some parents would prefer to be alone in the evenings anyway. It is always best to ask the parents what would be the most helpful to them. The experience of a new baby is different for each family, and they may have specific things that need to be done.

As Things Settle Down

Most doctors don't allow a woman to drive for two weeks after delivery—longer for a cesarian. This restriction can be difficult when she has a house to operate and family responsibilities. Offer to take the mom on her errands, or offer to do them for her. Even buying a roll of stamps can be a major production with a new baby.

The new mother may also become a bit stir-crazy in the house all day after being an active person who could pick up and go when she wanted. One woman related her shock the day she came home from the hospital with her first child and realized she would never be able to leave her house again without taking the child or making arrangements for her care.

Offer to stay with baby so Mom can enjoy a car ride or a trip to the espresso shop. Or baby-sit so the parents can go out for dinner or a movie. They need time together without the baby.

Bring in meals for the first few days. Cook enough so that there will be leftovers to reheat for another meal.

Call ahead to plan for a short visit, and be understanding if it's not a good time. Company is very important, but sometimes the baby's sleep periods are the only time parents can get anything done around the house; when the baby's awake she demands their full attention. If you can set a time to visit that is convenient to the parents, you will have a much more relaxing visit.

If you want to hold the baby during your visit, wash your hands first, as a simple courtesy and sanitary precaution. Don't ask to hold the baby if you are sick; in fact, wait to visit until you're over your bug. No one in the household needs to get sick at this time.

Don't forget the other children. Bring them a present when you bring one for the baby. Take them out for dinner or a special treat. The children will appreciate the attention, and the parents will appreciate time alone with the new baby.

Gift Ideas

Most gifts the family receives are for the baby and are very much appreciated, as babies are an expensive addition to the household. Layette items, clothes, strollers, swings, and furniture are all needed, especially for a first baby. Once the child is born, ask what the family still needs. It may be that there is a big-ticket item that several friends could purchase together.

Many moms mentioned how much they appreciated gifts for themselves.

- ❤ Chocolates for the new mom; a box of favorite candy
- ❤ A basket of bubble bath, bath powder, and other products for a relaxing bath
- ❤ Play clothes or casual wear in a larger size
- ❤ Gift certificates for personal care like hairstyling, pedicure, manicure, facial, or massage
- ❤ Gift certificates for a favorite restaurant, a play, or other special activity that the parents would enjoy. Offer to baby-sit.

- ♥ New negligée or peignoir set
- ♥ Diaper service for a day or week
- ♥ A visit from a house-cleaning service
- ♥ A coupon book of household tasks you are willing to do

In Closing

New families and families with new additions need lots of support during the weeks before and after the baby arrives.

What Can You Do to Help?

✓ Help the parents organize the house and nursery, so their full attention can be devoted to the baby when it comes home.

✓ Provide a special meal in the hospital, and bring in meals once the family gets home.

✓ Help with errands, shopping, and other household tasks that may be needed. Run a load of laundry, or tidy the house.

✓ Baby-sit so the parents can see a movie or go for a ride.

✓ Take the other children in the home out for a special activity, a movie, or a meal.

✓ Bring a gift to the new mom. She will appreciate being remembered.

Chapter Six

For Seriously, Chronically, or Terminally Ill Patients and for Those in Nursing Homes

People who live with chronic or terminal conditions or who require care in a nursing home need special attention and concern from friends and family. Regular contact is vital to the health and well-being of the patient. It is particularly important that the patient feel in touch with life outside the sickroom and that he be made to feel he is a part of the broader world. Families should ask his opinions on family matters whenever possible. Friends should keep him up to date on community life and local gossip.

Whether the condition has come on recently or has been with the person for his lifetime, the greatest gift you can give is to keep him an important part of your life.

Stay in Contact

Make an effort not to forget a person who is ill and not actively a part of your life. Put little notes in your personal calendar or on your desk to remind yourself to remember. It will be one of the most important things you do.

Send cards regularly. If the patient is unlikely to have a full recovery, adjust the card's message from "Get well soon" to "Thinking of you." One man with a terminal condition complained bitterly when he received cards with snappy little messages about a speedy recovery.

It may be helpful for you to plan a special time or circumstance when you visit—once a week with cookies, to watch a sporting event on television, or to watch a newly released video.

Hal brought doughnuts every Saturday morning to his neighbor with cancer and he would stay for a visit. The patient looked forward to Saturday and always seemed to have extra energy for Hal's visit.

If you set up a regular time to visit, be sure you keep it, or call to explain why you won't be there this week. People who are shut in are particularly pleased to have company, and they count on your regular visit. It can be very discouraging to wait for a friend who never arrives.

Visits from peers are important, as are visits from people of your same sex. Several men mentioned that they had primarily female caregivers and enjoyed seeing a male friend.

These are some other ways to remember:

- ❤ Send small care packages of fruit, nuts, special treats, or candy, if allowed. (Check diet restrictions.)
- ❤ Remember all holidays, not just Christmas. Don't forget Thanksgiving, Easter, the Fourth of July, Halloween, and birthdays. Even creating your own holiday—"Mary's Special Day"— is a way to bring fun to a person who is ill.
- ❤ Send a music cassette.
- ❤ Visit to watch a special sporting event or concert on television.
- ❤ Bring in a favorite meal or snack (if allowed).
- ❤ Tape a church service or a celebrity lecture and bring it to your friend. Stay so you can listen together.
- ❤ Loan CDs or tapes.
- ❤ Read a book, or arrange for books on tape.
- ❤ Bring fresh flowers each week. You'll need two vases, one to

leave and one for the next week. Arrange the flowers yourself.
- 💜 Send an audio letter.
- 💜 Read the headlines from the newspaper; clip interesting articles from papers and magazines.
- 💜 Order a subscription to a local paper so the patient can keep up with local news. This gift is particularly thoughtful if the patient has moved to another town for treatment or to be closer to family.

Organize a club, social, or church group to adopt shut-ins as secret pals and to send regular cards and small gifts.

Churches often establish committees responsible for care of shut-ins from the parish. In our church the committee members make regular visits to the shut-in. Each committee member is responsible for one or two people. He takes Christmas and birthday presents, sends regular cards, and makes sure the person's needs are being met. If a problem does arise, he can report it back to the committee and the minister for follow-up. Any social club can organize such a group. Friends can also organize themselves to take care of one of their own. Shared responsibility makes it easier to help.

The wife of a man who recently died after a long illness suggested that as a person's condition deteriorates, regular cards and notes are a better way to stay in touch than phone calls. Phone calls can be tiring, because the patient is required to keep up a conversation. He may feel that he has to say things like "I'm doing just great" when he doesn't feel like it. A card lets him know you're there, and he can read it when he feels up to it. If you aren't sure, ask a spouse or care-giver what would be best.

Make Life Easy

Look for ways to make the person's life easier, or provide him with tools to be as independent as possible. A wonderful idea for a person with limited mobility is to bring a "convenience basket." The basket includes things the patient will need close at hand: water canister, remote control, scissors, writing pad and pen, book or magazine, snacks of fruit, juice or cookies, crossword puzzle book, deck of cards and rules for solitaire, or other things the patient will use frequently. The basket can stay by the bed or travel with the patient from room to room.

Communicating may be difficult for the patient.

- ❤ Draft thank-you notes for the patient to sign.
- ❤ Offer to write out the letters he dictates.
- ❤ Provide a tape recorder so the patient can record his thoughts or create audio letters.
- ❤ Buy cards he can send to remember friends' special days.
- ❤ Give a portable phone as a gift.
- ❤ Dial the phone for calls the patient wants to make.

The patient will need a list of people who have written notes or sent presents. It will help him to decide how thank-yous will be handled.

Eating with dignity presents challenges to a patient who has restricted use of his hands or has trouble chewing or swallowing. Special silverware, straws, and other adaptive devices are available to help. The latest technology is available at a hospital supply store, which can also give you ideas for creative solutions to other problems the patient may face.

Housekeeping tasks in the sickroom are a concern whether the patient is at home, in a hospital, or in a nursing home. Straighten the patient's room periodically, and dust the furniture. It is important to the patient's morale that the sickroom be clean, smell fresh, and be visually appealing. Look for things that need to be done, and do them. Sometimes the thing that is most bothersome will not be apparent to a visitor. Ask the patient if there are any particular jobs he would like done.

Set up a regular time when you will help with tasks the patient can't do for himself. Make it a workable schedule for both you and the patient; for instance, one half hour to an hour a week. Even one errand is helpful.

Arrange the furniture so the most needed items are easily at hand. Put a table by the bed where he can stack things he will want to use again. Think through the design of the room to assure that items are efficiently and accessibly placed.

Creative Support Systems

There may be periods of time when the patient needs regular companionship or a specific kind of assistance. After chemotherapy or similar treatments, the patient may need someone at home for a few hours or overnight. He may not be able to drive or fix meals for a few days. To share the responsibility and give the patient the support he needs, organize a network of people who are available to help. Schedule the regular tasks so the patient knows what will be done and by whom, and provide a list of names and numbers for people willing to be on call for special assignments.

A group of friends arranged a schedule so one was always with a single friend when she went through chemotherapy. They took her to her appointment, stayed during the treatment, then spent the night at her home. This same kind of support could be provided for a person facing outpatient surgery or any type of regular medical treatment.

As people learned that we were writing this book, several made sure to tell us of a recent trend in which several hundred people join together to sustain and strengthen a friend with a terminal or chronic illness. These support systems provide regular calls, letters, and help to the patient and work with him toward recovery, remission, or a positive quality of life. They provide a list of people to call if he feels down, and designate boosters who let him know how valuable he is to them.

One group, Linda's Lifeguards, formed when Linda, age thirty-three, was diagnosed with leukemia. The Lifeguards ran errands, baby-sat, wrote her regularly, and prayed for her. Friends of friends from around the country were added until the list numbered over 1,000. Shortly before her death, Linda was quoted in the *Chicago*

Tribune as saying, "Never once have I felt alone in this. How could I when I have such an incredible team rallied behind me? Every cancer patient needs a team like this."

Support groups of this kind offer tremendous emotional support to the patient and give him a reason to live. They also provide the helpers with a wonderful opportunity to grow spiritually through the experience of helping another person. You'll also meet some other special people along the way. Select a name that symbolizes help and hope, like the Lifeguards, Guardian Angels, or Bear Cats. Prepare buttons for all the helpers or T-shirts that announce that you are part of the group. Make it a positive activity for all involved.

Improve the Patient's Living Space

The world can feel like it's closing in when you're confined to just a few rooms. It's easy to become bored and lose interest in life. One way to improve a person's attitude is to improve his physical surroundings.

- ❤ Paint the room a new color, or put up wallpaper, if the patient agrees. The patient should choose colors and patterns.
- ❤ Move the furniture to create a different view.
- ❤ Find ways to personalize the room with family pictures, favorite figurines, or other personal mementos. Put a collage of pictures of family and friends on the wall, and change them periodically.
- ❤ Use posters and inexpensive decorations to create themes for the room, and change them regularly. Seasons, holidays, animals,

movies, elections, or special interests are all decorating ideas the patient might enjoy.

💜 Fix things that do not work in the room or are an eyesore. Put a slipcover on an old chair, wash the curtains, or clean the windows.

💜 Change pictures, artwork, and other decorations on a regular basis.

💜 Keep the room smelling fresh with potpourri and scented candles.

💜 Clean up the yard or the view out the window.

Bring the Outdoors Inside

There is something calming about nature; it gives people a feeling of peace and renewal. If the patient can't leave his room or go outside on a regular basis, look for ways to bring the outside to him.

💜 Through posters, paintings, and plants you can create a feeling of nature in the room.

💜 Hang a bird feeder by the bedroom window so it is seen from the patient's bed. Be sure to keep it filled with food. Give him a book about backyard birds so that he can identify the different birds that come to the feeder. Videos on songbirds are also available.

💜 Rent nature videos and materials on animals, parks, or other nature subjects, or borrow them from the library. Decorate the room with posters of similar sights.

- Bring in fresh flowers and plants regularly, if the patient's condition permits. Blooming plants are most colorful. If fresh plants are not allowed, try silk plants; they are so lifelike today that it's hard to tell that they aren't real.
- Set up an aquarium in the room. Provide background information on the different species of fish in the tank.
- Birds also make cheerful pets for shut-ins, if other animals in the house don't object.
- Prepare a window garden, or plant seeds in small containers for transplant outside when the weather permits.

Move Outside Whenever Possible

Find ways the patient can be outside, even for a limited time. Fresh air is healing.

- Take a short walk, even just in front of the house or building. It will give the patient a feeling of freedom.
- Use a wheelchair to take him for a walk if mobility is a problem.
- A car ride can provide a much-needed break.
- Provide a chair so the patient can sit outside the door if he can go no farther. The idea is fresh air and a change of scenery; time and distance don't matter.
- On a warm summer day, create a place to rest on a porch or in a shaded area under a tree.

Create Surprises

Make life interesting by creating surprises.
- ❤ Invent a special reason to have a celebration— "It's Monday!"
- ❤ Visit wearing a mask or costume for Halloween or another time.
- ❤ Tape recorded messages from friends. Take Polaroid pictures while they are making the recording, then display the photos in the sickroom.
- ❤ Arrange for a special friend or relative, perhaps someone from out of town who hasn't seen the patient for some time, to visit.
- ❤ Organize special friends or buddies, a group that has hung out together in the past, to visit and play cards or another game they enjoy. Watch a movie or a sports event together.
- ❤ Arrange for a hairstylist, barber, or manicurist to make a visit to the patient.

If the patient is in a nursing home or other extended-care facility, hire a barbershop quartet or Sweet Adelines to entertain for all the patients. Play the piano for a singalong, or find someone who will. Bring well-trained animals to visit, or have an amateur group perform a short play.

Celebrate Life

Celebrate the patient's life while he is alive. Let him know that he matters to you and that you will always treasure the times you have shared together.

Create a scrapbook with the story of the person's life in pictures and articles. His family can help locate photographs for the book and you can hold a *This is Your Life*-type evening when you give the patient the book and discuss the high points in his life.

If the patient is a saver, he may have boxes of mementos. Ask him if you can go through the boxes together—you will learn a lot about him, and you may find some treasures that can be preserved or displayed.

Produce a living history by asking the patient to tell you about the changes he has experienced in his life, and record the conversation on an audio- or videotape. Not only will the tape be an important legacy for the family, but it will let the patient know how important his life has been.

One family asked their grandmother to talk on an audiotape about all the changes she had seen in her lifetime, from her childhood when transportation was a horse and buggy to the men landing on the moon. What a treasure this family will have for generations to come! One by-product of this project was that the children took a greater interest in history and did research on their own.

Create a scrapbook of special times you shared together. School, work, or family memories can be assembled from your personal collection of pictures and souvenirs. What a nice surprise, especially if you have pictures the patient hasn't seen for many years.

Write the patient a letter telling him how important he has been in your life and how much you have appreciated his friendship.

Arrange a special event to honor the person who is ill. Invite friends who have known the person a long time or have shared common experiences. If a large event would be too tiring, invite small groups. Allow for opportunities to celebrate the person while he is alive.

In one case a close friend arranged a special tribute to his dying friend. Family and old friends came from across the country to be a part of the evening. They dined in a private dining room; then each friend toasted and roasted the honored guest. The evening was videotaped and provided hours of pleasure after the event as well. It also meant a great deal to the family left behind.

Seek out old school chums, family who live far away, and other friends who may have wandered away over the years, so they can get in touch while the patient is well enough to hear from them.

Organize a reunion of school friends or college classmates. We learned of six college friends who traveled to California from all parts of the country to support a classmate who was dying of cancer. They exchanged funny gifts, wrote poems, meditated together, and cooked a turkey banquet. They laughed a lot and thoroughly enjoyed each other's company. They took lots of photos and made scrapbooks for their friend and for themselves, so they could relive the weekend in pictures. One member of the group had the group's picture made into a calendar for each person.

Arrange for a family reunion over the holidays. Help those who may have financial difficulties to attend, if you can afford it. Decide to forgo holiday presents, and use the money to come together for the reunion.

Nothing you do will be more rewarding than making the effort to be with a person while he is still alive. If you have the money to visit only once, do it now, not for his funeral. He will appreciate it more!

Other Ideas When the Patient Is Terminal

There are many programs that grant special requests to dying patients. Most are for children, but some include adults as well. Look into these programs for the family of the terminal patient; find out the criteria for participation and how applications are made. Give the family the information you find, and help them follow through. You will provide a valuable service and save the family members hours of research at a time when they have other pressing demands.

Often you can write to the patient's favorite celebrity to ask for a letter or autographed picture. Sometimes a celebrity who is scheduled to be in the area will meet with the patient. A woman in our community who was terminally ill loved Reba McIntyre and wanted to see her at a scheduled concert in town. Although she was terribly ill, she went to the concert and visited Reba in her dressing room. She received a personally autographed picture and, according to her family, was thrilled to see her favorite star. She died the next morning.

Call a radio disc jockey and send a special hello to the patient, or ask a local columnist to recognize the person for a special achievement he made in his life. Use local celebrities to assist with fund-raising programs on the patient's behalf. For a full discussion of fund-raising events, see chapter 11.

If the patient is a fan of a sports team, arrange for the coach to visit or for the team to send an autographed ball. In some cases the team will dedicate the game to a fan or give him the game ball.

You may want to help the family contact a hospice program as well as other organizations in your community that help in these situations. Be sure, however, that the family is ready. Once I offered to contact the hospice program for a friend whose husband was dying. She assured me that the program was only for people who were terminal and not something that she and her husband needed. Her husband died two weeks later.

Gift Ideas

- ♥ New nightclothes
- ♥ Comfortable clothes—lightweight sweatshirts and sweatpants
- ♥ VCR: Loan one to the patient, or purchase it if your funds permit
- ♥ Favorite videos—new releases or classics
- ♥ Picture books
- ♥ Prints or posters for the wall
- ♥ CDs and tapes
- ♥ Books on tape
- ♥ Video travelogues
- ♥ Collage of photos
- ♥ Scrapbook

- ❤ Table that can fit over the bed
- ❤ An insulated coffee cup with a screw-on top that keeps a beverage hot for a long time and won't cause a spill if it is accidentally knocked over
- ❤ Gifts of laughter—humor books, old slapstick movies and television shows, or classic radio tapes

If the patient's condition is improving, and there is hope for recovery, send gifts that look toward the future: golf balls, gardening tools, passes for cross-country skiing.

In Closing

Special efforts must be made to include a patient who has a serious, chronic, or terminal condition or who is confined to a nursing home. He needs to feel a part of his family, community, and group of friends.

What Can You Do to Help?

- ✓ By whatever means you have available, stay in contact with the patient. Include him in family decisions, and let him know his contributions are valued.
- ✓ Look for ways to make the patient's life easier. Help with tasks that need to be done, and provide him with the tools to be as independent as possible.

✓ Organize a support system of friends, coworkers, and members of organizations to which the patient belongs. Even friends of friends can participate. Have this support system provide tangible help like cards, phone calls, and visits. Be on call if the patient needs special assistance or a listening ear.

✓ Improve the place where the patient lives through decorations, pictures, and upkeep.

✓ Integrate nature and the out-of-doors into the patient's life through the addition of natural settings to his room. Try to move him outside, if only for a short period of time.

✓ Celebrate the person's life while he is alive. If you can only visit once, do it while he is living. Bring him tokens that let him know how much he is appreciated.

Chapter Seven

Remembering the Siblings and Children

When a parent, brother, or sister is ill, the other children in the home are also affected. Their natural need for order and security is compromised. Parents are preoccupied (perhaps at the hospital), meals become irregular, caregivers vary and may even be strangers, and the children are often left to try to understand more than their limited experience will allow.

Friends and relatives can step in at this time and can provide much needed support to the children and the parents.

Maintaining a Normal Life

The healthy child still has her life, activities, and problems, which continue regardless of family circumstances. Any assistance you can offer to maintain her normal life with as few disruptions as possible will make the situation easier on everyone involved. Help her attend her usual activities by driving her to swim lessons, play practice, or soccer games. Wash uniforms or iron costumes so she can participate fully.

It may be appropriate to involve her in more activities than usual, so that she spends time with children her own age and is not dependent on her home for entertainment. Outside activities will also take her mind off the situation at home. It is important the child not feel she is being sent away, dismissed, or punished. She should be included in all decisions involving additional activities.

If it is summer, enroll her in a day camp or other special programs that are offered by museums, churches, nature centers, or local colleges. There are football camps, basketball camps, drama camps, church camps, computer camps, and camps for many other interests the child may have. If the enrollment period has passed, ask the organizers if spots are still available. It may be possible for the child to register late, especially if the circumstances are explained. One family enrolled their child in a day camp operated by the local YWCA. While it was intended for the children of working parents, it provided great daily activities for the child while her father was in the hospital.

During the school year, many after-school activities are offered. School officials will usually know of programs that are available and will work with the family on registration and transportation. Teachers and counselors at the healthy child's school should be kept fully informed of the family situation. They will likely have experience in dealing with similar situations and can offer help in arranging activities, suggesting alternatives, and working with the family if the child must miss school. In addition, counselors and teachers can help the child work through her emotions about the situation at home.

Jessica's grade-school counselor made a special effort to check in with her on a regular basis. The counselor was able to talk with Jessica about her worries and to offer guidance at a critical time, letting Jessica know that another adult was there for her.

It is helpful for someone to be home when the child returns from school. She will need to satisfy herself that everything is all right there and that nothing has changed while she's been away. She may also want to talk about her day and to ask questions about her family situation.

If it is not possible for a parent or family member to be at home, or if the family is at the hospital, a friend who lives nearby may be willing to have the child come to her home after school. A familiar face will provide security in uncertain times.

Lauren was willing to be at home every day when her neighbors' son was in the hospital. Their other son, Jason, came to her house for a snack and to play after school, and then other family members picked him up for dinner. Jason really enjoyed going to Lauren's and knowing there was some regular routine in his life.

Keeping the circle of friends and playmates intact is also important. The situation at home may not allow the healthy child to invite friends in to play, so a plan should be made for her to visit friends' houses to play, for sleepovers, and to be a part of other group activities.

Keeping classwork current should also be a top priority. Help the child with her school homework, piano practice, or science project so she doesn't fall behind. The child is already under pressure from the disruption at home; she doesn't need the added stress of falling behind in school.

Creating an Honest Environment

When children are not given facts and full explanations of family situations, their fertile imaginations make them up. It is amazing what stories will emerge from a child who has developed her own conclusions about a set of circumstances.

When Jessica was told that Nicholas was going to the hospital, she believed he would die. The two people she knew who had gone into a hospital, a grandfather and an aunt, had both died, so it was a logical conclusion in her mind that Nicholas would meet the same fate. It was important that she have the opportunity to express her fears so that the basis of those fears could be specifically addressed.

Don't think you are sparing the child from worry by keeping the situation secret; in reality she will worry more because of the explanations her mind creates. She will likely feel that things must be really bad if no one will tell her what's going on, or she may blame herself for both the illness and the secrecy.

Tell the truth in terms the child can understand. If at all possible take the child to visit the family member in the hospital. Hospitals may seem like scary places to a child whose only association is with older relatives who go in and never come out. When she can see things for herself, she will be less frightened and more willing to work with parents and other caregivers during the crisis.

As circumstances change in the course of the illness, be sure the child is given the new information and regular progress reports. She should be given as much information as she can understand.

Once our lives returned to some degree of normalcy and Jessica had gone home to stay, I asked the parents for a full briefing on Nick's condition. While I knew all the basics, I had no technical background, as I had always been with Jessica when things were explained, so the information I had was at a seven-year-old level.

If alternative arrangements must be made for the child's care, she should participate in the decision and have some choices if at all possible. She may have a preference about which relative cares for her, and will be happier if those preferences can be honored.

In the first few days after Nicholas entered the hospital, many friends and relatives offered to care for Jessica and invited her to the movies or other activities. She seemed in conflict about these invitations, not sure what we wanted her to do or whether she should accept an invitation even if she didn't want to. We created "Jessica gets to do whatever she wants" days, and she was allowed to decide which of the invitations, if any, she accepted. In this way she felt comfortable stating her preferences and didn't feel the family was trying to get rid of her.

It is also important to create a safe environment where the healthy child can ask questions and express her feelings and emotions. Let her speak freely, and respect her point of view. She should never be made to feel stupid or silly. She may have misinformation that needs to be corrected, but it should always be done in an environment of love and understanding.

If the child has trouble expressing herself or seems reluctant to share her thoughts, provide some vehicle that will allow her to give voice to her concerns and fears. Journals and puppets are often used to help children express themselves. Be supportive, understanding, and honest. Don't ever laugh or dismiss her pain; what may seem funny through our adult eyes is very real to a child. She will keep silent if she fears ridicule.

Give the Healthy Child a Role

The healthy child should have a role in helping the family cope with the illness. Maybe she can take on additional household duties, such as doing the dishes or mowing the lawn. These should be jobs that are not currently her responsibility. She needs to know she is being asked to do them to help out; then her contribution needs to be acknowledged.

Emily learned to mow the lawn when her father was in the hospital. She was very proud of the job she did, showing it off to everyone who visited, and she felt herself a part of the family in a more important way than she had in the past; she was no longer a dependent child but a contributor.

When the healthy child must give up an activity because no one can take her to it or because it would interfere with other more pressing matters, her sacrifice should be acknowledged, even with just a thank you. She should feel that her cooperation in forgoing her activity is appreciated, even if she wasn't too willing to give it up at first.

Encourage her to make something for her sibling who is ill—a card, a picture—or to write a story. Jessica wrote Nicholas a story the first morning he was in the hospital. When she went to visit she read it to him, which gave them an opportunity to do something together.

Remembering

When one child is very ill most of the attention is naturally directed there, leaving the healthy child on her own. When visiting the child who is ill, make an effort to include and remember the healthy child. Bring her a small gift when you visit her brother or sister who is ill. It doesn't have to be of the same value, just a symbol to let the child know she is remembered and valued. It also conveys to both children that you don't have to be sick to get presents.

Include the healthy child in the life of your family. If you are eating out or going to a movie, invite her to join you. Include her in family picnics, outings to the beach, or in other activities you have planned. If her sibling or parent is seriously ill, there may be few special outings in her family for a while.

Send her a card now and then, or call and ask how she is getting along.

Creating Special Times

Special memories can be created out of a difficult situation. Look for opportunities to do something just for her, or take her to new places.

When Nicholas was in the hospital, Jessica spent two weeks in California with Buffy's brother and his family. The parents were able to focus their full attention on Nicholas, and Jessica had a break from the family situation and a chance to see places she had never seen before. She also built a bond with her cousins that will last a lifetime.

Invite the healthy child to spend a night or weekend at your house. Children love to visit. Take her on a day or overnight trip. Spend the night in a local hotel with a pool. Some hotels have poolside rooms and cater to families with children, with special toys and recreation areas.

Help the child plan for the future. Make a list of things she'd like to do when family life returns to normal. Give her a piggy bank to use in saving for a special treat when her sibling recovers. Help the children plan the way they will use the money raised to celebrate.

You can share any number of activities with the healthy child. Take her to a sports event, the zoo, an amusement park, a hands-on museum, or a children's fun house. Fly a kite.

Lunch or dinner out can be a treat, especially at her favorite restaurant.

Give her a chance just to spend time with you—even running errands or fixing a meal can be fun as a change of pace.

Ask parents or other family what things you could do with the child that would also be a service to the parents. Some ideas might include shopping for school clothes or a relative's birthday present, or helping her clean and organize her room. These activities will help you get to know the child in a relaxed setting and may provide additional ideas for things you can do together.

In Closing

The healthy child will have a range of emotions, questions, and conflicts when someone in her family becomes ill. Attention will be diverted from her, and the foundation of her life may feel shaky.

What Can You Do to Help?

✓ Keep her life as normal as possible by maintaining the family routine and by encouraging her to participate in her regular activities. Facilitate that involvement by providing transportation, lunch, clean clothes, or whatever else is needed.

✓ Tell the truth about the illness, and about changes that may occur in the family, in terms the child can understand. Don't ignore the child's questions or assume the child is too young to comprehend the situation. In fact, if she doesn't receive satisfactory answers, she'll likely make some up that will be far more frightening than the truth.

✓ Look for ways the child can help during the illness. Create a role that allows her to make a positive contribution to family life, and thank her for sacrifices she may make along the way.

✓ Don't forget the healthy child when you bring a present to the child that is ill. A small package of stickers or a new game will make the healthy child feel important.

✓ Look for opportunities to include and involve the healthy child in your life. Create special memories together.

Chapter Eight

Caring for the Caregiver

Illness has a way of striking when a family is least prepared. The laundry isn't done, the dishes are in the kitchen sink, and the children's toys are spread throughout the house. Yet there is no time to put things in order—an emergency is at hand. These are the moments when family and close friends can save the day.

When our mother suffered a sudden heart attack in the middle of the night, my sister's in-laws arrived the next morning, cleaned every room, made the beds with fresh linen, did all the laundry, and fixed a large stew that lasted several days. The relief we felt when we arrived home that night was overwhelming.

Stepping In

In the first few hours or days of an illness, everyday tasks are lost. If you want to be of help in the early hours of an illness emergency, you may find the most critical tasks to be done involve housekeeping.

- ❤ Unload the dishwasher, or do any dishes collecting in the sink.
- ❤ Straighten the house. It's not necessary to put things away, and it may not be a good idea since you might have a different idea of where things should go. Just make neat piles the family can go through when they have time.
- ❤ Cook a hot meal—something that will last and can be heated up without harm, like stews, chili, or casseroles.
- ❤ Answer the phone and take messages. A list with name, number, and message will make it easy for the family to return calls.

Include the date and time, as it may be days before the call is returned.

- Loan the family a telephone answering machine if they don't have one. It will be a lifesaver.
- Run a load of laundry. You may want to skip personal items if you choose, but sheets, towels, and everyday clothes are always needed.
- Put fresh linens on the beds, or at least make them so the beds are ready when the weary family returns. There is something so inviting about a freshly made bed after a long day at the hospital.
- Empty wastepaper baskets, and take out the trash. Move trash cans to the curb on trash pickup day.
- Water plants.
- Mow the lawn, or shovel the snow.
- Bring in mail and newspapers.

Mary stepped in when a neighbor's father went into the hospital. She trimmed the flowers in the garden, weeded the vegetable plants, and tended the garden throughout the summer. The family was very grateful to have their garden cared for all summer.

If there are young children or pets in the home, some arrangements must be made for their care. Depending on the nature of the illness and its duration, the family may just need someone to watch over them for the day, or may need a more long-term solution.

Family or friends who are able to take small children or pets for a few days can ease a tremendous burden.

Alice's mother wrote me that when her daughter was seriously ill, her neighbor canned all her tomatoes, and the neighbor's husband kept the lawn mowed. "She never asked what needed to be done; she just did what was needed to be done." She added, "My brother and sister-in-law took our two-year-old boy. If not for them, I don't know how we would have made it. We needed to focus all our attention on Alice, and that allowed us to do it."

Another immediate task the family faces is informing family and friends of the situation. If you are willing to make calls, ask the family whom they would like you to contact. Don't make calls on your own, there may be people they would prefer to contact personally. Once you've agreed on the list, make the calls you are assigned, and keep the list for follow-up.

Keep a list of all the cards, gifts, and food that is received so the family can properly acknowledge the helpers.

It's the Thought that Counts

You may not feel you know the family well enough to take over personal needs, or you may not be in a position to commit to ongoing involvement over an extended period of time. There are many other ways you can provide support and help.

Don't underestimate the power of a greeting card, short note, or small gift specifically for the caregiver. Many families who were responsible for the care of sick relatives mentioned how much it meant to hear from friends. The caregivers are often unsung and forgotten heroes. It means a great deal when their contribution is recognized.

Phone calls have the same effect. If you are at home all day caring for a sick child or parent, a call from a friend can provide a much-needed break. Don't worry about interrupting; just ask when you call if this is a convenient time to talk. Set a better time to call back if your friend can't talk at that moment.

It may be that you haven't been in contact for a long time and feel uncomfortable calling after so much time has passed. Chances are that your friend will be thrilled to hear from you and touched that you would be so thoughtful as to remember him at a difficult time.

If you would like to do more, you may ask the family directly what would be helpful, but don't give up if they say they're fine— especially if it is clear that they are not.

A close friend or relative may know what is needed. Ask him for ideas, or suggest something you would like to do, and ask if that would be appropriate.

The Gift of Time

Often the most thoughtful gift for the caregiver is time—time to get away, time to renew himself, time to think of something beyond his immediate situation.

If you know the patient and are willing to spend time in the sickroom, offer to sit with him while the caregiver takes a break, even if it is just to take a shower or go to an exercise class. An hour can mean a lot. An evening out is even better.

Be specific: "What night can I come and stay so you can go to a movie?" or "I'll sit here for a few minutes, and you go to the cafeteria and have some lunch."

If your schedule allows, set a consistent time each day or week that you will visit to give the caregiver a break he can count on. Fresh company will also give the patient a boost.

A gift certificate is another thoughtful way to give time and can be used at the caregiver's convenience. Gift certificates are available for most activities, including:

- ❤ Movies
- ❤ Personal care items such as a hairstyling, massage, pedicure, or manicure
- ❤ Tickets to shows, concerts, sporting events, or other special programs
- ❤ Overnight at a favorite hotel or bed and breakfast
- ❤ Dinner at a favorite restaurant
- ❤ Time in a hot tub
- ❤ Court time or greens fees for a favorite sport
- ❤ Miniature golf

You may offer to stay with the patient or pay the baby-sitter, but it is not a requirement. A gift of time is appropriate even if the caregiver has to make some arrangements.

A visit to the caregiver can be a valuable gift of time. You can help him take his mind off his problems, or you can be a listening ear—whichever is needed. Set a date to exercise together or to have lunch. The caregiver needs diversion as much as the patient, maybe more.

When the Caregiver Must Stay at the Hospital

When the patient is a small child or is critically ill, the primary caregiver often must spend hours at the hospital. In some circumstances he may not leave for days at a time. In these situations, the caregiver needs support and contact with the outside world. Here are some ways you can reach out:

- ❤ Prepare a favorite dish or sandwich.
- ❤ Bring in lunch or dinner from a favorite restaurant.
- ❤ Bring a change of clothes or toiletries.
- ❤ Drop off soda and snacks.
- ❤ Sit with the patient so the caregiver can run an errand or even can go home for an hour or two.
- ❤ Bring magazines or a book. Choose the caregiver's favorite authors or subject, and be sure the subject is not too heavy or requiring of deep thought. He is doing enough thinking already. Mysteries, Westerns, and Romances are great in this situation.
- ❤ Bring videos, if equipment is available, or loan a VCR and a few favorite tapes.
- ❤ It is a good idea to visit in pairs. One person can stay with the patient while the other goes for a walk or to the cafeteria with the caregiver.

When one child required a lengthy hospitalization, we prepared fresh sandwiches for the parents each day. It was a nice break for them, and it provided a meal they were more likely to eat, as it was quick and to their tastes. Occasionally we brought the couple dinner from their favorite restaurant—Chinese one night, Mexican the next—anything to break the monotony and give the parents a change from the hospital menu. A small bottle of wine can also help the parents relax, if they are people who would appreciate the gesture.

More Long-term Needs

If the illness is expected to continue for any period of time, you may wish to organize ongoing support for the family through a network of friends or an organization. In our church a committee is organized to provide dinner for families with medical emergencies. Each person who participates agrees to bring dinner one night, and the family is provided a schedule of whom to expect and when. In this way the responsibility for preparing meals is shared among the group, and the worry of feeding the family is removed from the caregiver.

If you wish to organize this kind of support, establish a schedule. When people ask if they can bring a meal, assign them a convenient night. Give the family the schedule, with phone numbers, so they will know who to expect and can make contact directly if changes are needed.

These are other things that can help the caregiver.

♥ Buy groceries, especially staples. With eggs, milk, and bread in the house, you can always make a meal.

- ❤ Mow the lawn, shovel the snow, or rake leaves on a regular basis to keep the yard attractive.
- ❤ Take small appliances to be repaired.
- ❤ Run other errands.
- ❤ Take or pick up dry cleaning.
- ❤ Take the children gift shopping if a birthday or other special day is coming up.
- ❤ Transport a relative or friend for a visit, or pick up incoming family from the airport.
- ❤ Offer visiting family a room in your home.
- ❤ Keep the mail.

Consider the things you do to keep your own home running. These may be tasks that would be helpful to a family in crisis.

One clever way of offering help is to prepare a coupon book of things you or your group are willing to do, for instance, mow the lawn, shop for groceries, patient-sit, lunch out, pet care. The caregiver can then "redeem" the coupons for those tasks that would be most helpful. Include a few blank coupons the caregiver can make out for things you may not have considered.

If the patient has a serious illness, or if the family faces several issues that need to be addressed, compile a list, with phone numbers and addresses, of local community organizations that assist families in similar situations. Being able to make the necessary contacts without having to search through the phone book can be an important time-saver to an already stressed person.

Another important function is keeping friends and coworkers informed of progress, the patient's condition, and new needs that may arise.

The Family Pet

Pets can be another concern, especially if the illness takes the family away from home for long days.

- ❤ Offer to take the dog for a walk, once or daily if your schedule permits.
- ❤ Arrange for a neighbor child to come in each day and walk the dog. You will need to pay a small nominal fee for that service, but it will mean a great deal to the family. You can also pay for one week and then let the family pick it up from there, if they are interested.
- ❤ Change the cat's litter box.
- ❤ Feed the guinea pig and change its water.
- ❤ Feed the fish, and leave a note that you have done it.
- ❤ Consider taking the animal to your home, if it is appropriate and agreeable to the caregiver.

Buffy's brother took her dog home when Nicholas was first in the hospital. It was such a relief to know that the dog was safe and receiving proper care.

It may be necessary to board the dog or cat in a kennel until things are more settled. You can offer to make the arrangements and transport the pet, but the caregiver and family must make the decision that the animal is to be boarded. The pet may offer solace to the family, and they may prefer that it stay in the home.

In Closing

It is the caregiver who often shoulders the major responsibility in a family illness, not only caring for the patient, but also keeping the household running and family life as normal as possible.

What Can You Do to Help?

✓ Chances are that the illness struck with little warning or time to prepare. Step in to help with household tasks and errands that may need to be done immediately.

✓ Take the children and pets to your home for a day or so, until the situation sorts itself out and more permanent arrangements can be made.

✓ Send cards, visit, and phone. Let the caregiver know he is not forgotten.

✓ Offer to stay with the patient so the caregiver can get away for a short time. Give other gifts of time, so the caregiver can get away from the situation to relax and renew.

✓ Don't forget the pets in the home. They can't take care of themselves when the family is away.

✓ As time goes on, stay in touch and help with household responsibilities, yard work, transportation, or other tasks that would be helpful to the caregiver on an ongoing basis.

Chapter Nine

Tips for a Successful Visit

L et's face it: visiting a hospital is seldom fun. Even if you are there for a happy reason, such as the birth of a child, other people you encounter are most likely dealing with a serious health situation.

Some of us fear hospitals. We are concerned we might catch something from one of the patients, or that we might see blood or people who are disfigured. We also worry that the patient may be in pain or sick to her stomach and that we might be expected to help.

Chances are some of these things might happen, but most are unlikely. The critically ill and injured are normally in intensive care units or in an isolation that keeps them from public view. There are, however, sick people in a hospital—no question about it. You have to be truly sick to spend a night in a hospital.

If You Don't Feel You Can Visit—Don't!

If visiting a patient at the hospital is beyond what you personally can handle, don't go. The last thing a patient needs is to spend her time worrying about you. Tell the truth: "Mary, I'd love to come and see you, but I don't do well in hospitals. I'll be the first one to visit when you get home."

By being honest you don't raise false expectations, and you don't have to feel guilty. If you say you will visit and don't, you leave the patient waiting for you, perhaps cleaning up each day in anticipation of your arrival, and you feel like scum every day you don't show up. The guilt may also keep you away when your friend comes home and could drive a permanent wedge in your relationship.

There is no law that says you have to visit. Send a card, flowers, or balloons, or do any of the household tasks recommended in this book. Any thoughtful gesture will let her know you are thinking of her. She will appreciate flowers in her room far more than having you nauseated and complaining about the hospital smells.

Making Your Visit Count

If you are up for it and the patient's condition permits, by all means visit. Hospital days start early and last a long time. The patient's day will likely involve lying in bed all day and watching stupid television programs, reading old magazines, and staring at the four walls while being poked, prodded, tested, and retested. It can be a dreary existence.

The patient usually wants company, and hospitals encourage it. That's why there are visiting hours. Visiting hours are designated for a specific purpose; they are the most convenient time for you to visit. Usually baths, tests, and other assorted hospital activities are out of the way before visiting hours begin. Except in the case of an extremely unusual situation, you should always adhere to the visiting hours set by the hospital.

While visiting hours give you the times to visit, the patient's condition should dictate exactly when to visit. Just after surgery or the birth of a child, it may not be appropriate for those outside the immediate family to call on the patient. By the next day, however, guests may be very welcome. When in doubt, check with the family.

One woman who had major abdominal surgery was visited by her boss the morning after her surgery, when she was still groggy and in a hospital nightgown. He wanted her opinion as an outsider about a work situation in which she wasn't even involved. Needless to say, that was one visit she could have done without.

Why Are You There?

This brings us to the purpose of your visit, which should be to give comfort to the patient. If you have any other reason for being there, don't go.

A hospital visit, or any visit to a person who is ill, is not a social occasion. Keep the conversation light, and stay only a brief time; ten to fifteen minutes is sufficient unless the patient is very energetic. As soon as the patient seems to fade out of the conversation, closes her eyes, or yawns, you should know it is time to leave.

You may have come a long way, and you may hate to leave after only ten minutes. Leave anyway; you are there for the patient. In this situation, have lunch or a cup of coffee, and come back. Give the patient a chance to rest. Two short visits will mean more than one long stay, particularly if the patient tires easily.

Do not visit the hospital if you do not feel well. Again, why are you visiting? If you are only trying to be a good person, forget it. The patient will have much kinder thoughts of you if you don't give her the flu while she is trying to recover from surgery. Here again, be honest and explain why you aren't able to visit. She will understand and appreciate your thoughtfulness.

Keep It Light

Most people who are ill feel lousy; that's how they know they're sick. It is hard, when you feel horrid, to be pleasant and keep up a fast-paced conversation. If the patient seems cranky, angry, or down-right hostile when you visit, try to ignore it. She is not herself. Don't take it personally. If she seems to have a legitimate complaint, see if you can help.

Come prepared with a few topics you can discuss to keep the conversation moving. Harmless gossip the patient might enjoy, such as engagements or funny stories from work, news from mutual friends or family members, movies or concerts you have seen, or whatever will be interesting but will not require her to make decisions or talk too much, are good topics. She should not be the one who has to think of things to say.

Bring a current magazine with general interest stories or a crossword puzzle book you can leave behind. That way the patient has something to do if she is alone later in the day.

Don't share family problems or work conflicts or ask her to take sides in disputes. The hospital is not the place to iron out differences. We heard of one case in which warring family members came at the same time to visit their grandmother and argued the whole time they were in her room. She was sicker when they left than before they came, and it took her days to recover from the stress of the visit.

Malicious gossip has no place in the hospital either; it may upset the patient for no good reason. There will be plenty of time to share such information when the patient is well, if you must.

Another don't involves fragrances—don't wear heavy perfume or cologne when you visit. Strong odors can turn a fragile stomach.

She Knows She's Sick

Often we feel the need to say something that will help the patient feel better about her situation. We say things like "You're going to be just fine" or "There is nothing to worry about." Try to resist the temptation. Unless you are a doctor, you don't have adequate knowledge to be offering opinions on medical matters. Period. The patient knows she is sick and likely knows how sick she is. In an earlier time, patients were often spared the facts of their condition, but not today. If an illness is terminal the patient knows it. She needs your support and comfort; she doesn't need friends telling her she will be just fine when she knows she won't. Sadly, we make these hopeful comments because it is difficult for us to face the fact that a friend is dying. It is really our own need for comfort, rather than hers, that drives these comments, and if we aren't careful we will have the patient trying to make us feel better!

Before you arrive try to accept in your own mind the diagnosis and prognosis. Once you can come to grips with the inevitability of the situation, you can put aside your needs and concentrate on the patient. After all, she is the one dying.

There is no need to offer any opinion about the patient's prognosis or how she may be feeling. Simply say, "It's good to see you sitting in a chair today" or "You seem more alert today; are you feeling better?" That last question does not presume anything about the patient's condition, but rather allows her to tell you how she is feeling. Looks can be deceiving; a smile can hide a lot of discomfort.

Sharing Related Experiences

We can get into dangerous waters by sharing information with the patient about someone we knew with a similar condition. Why is it that when an acquaintance begins a story about someone they knew with a similar affliction, it always turns out that the person died? When it comes to information about her illness, let the patient direct the conversation. It may be very helpful to talk about how she is feeling and about her general condition. If she knows your brother had a similar disease, and wants to know about it, she will ask. Much of what we know about our illnesses we learn from others who have faced the same situation. The point is to share factual information that will be helpful to the patient, not to say things that might scare her unnecessarily.

If she wants to talk about her illness, let her. Terminal patients say that one of their most difficult challenges is wanting to discuss their condition and having no one who will listen. People change the subject or leave the room rather than listen to a dying friend talk about her illness.

Be careful not to bad-mouth the patient's doctor. Her confidence in her physician is none of your business. If your reservations are serious or come from personal experience, share them with the immediate family, and let them decide if there is anything to do.

Bottom Line: Think before You Speak

In our society we have developed a series of things we say when someone is ill and we don't know what else to say. A few favorites include "God never gives us more than we can handle." "When one door closes another opens." "You look so well." "Life goes on."

While these statements are offered as sincere words of comfort and encouragement, our research found that they universally upset the patient. They trivialize her genuine pain and dismiss the distress she may feel at the time.

My friend Judy told us of a doctor who called the parents of a sick child one night to tell them they needed to get on with their lives. "Life goes on," he stated, apparently pronouncing a death sentence on the child, who had been in the hospital several weeks with no concrete diagnosis. The parents were devastated, then angry. How dare he feel they could have a life if they lost their precious daughter?

Rather than offering a phrase that shuts off conversation, ask the patient about her illness and let her tell you where she is getting her strength. Her answers may guide you to a response that will address more directly what she is feeling. For instance, you may ask, "Has the surgery made you feel better?" "Has the doctor mentioned if special assistance will be needed when you get home?" "How are you feeling about your diagnosis?" "What has the doctor said about your prognosis?" These types of questions let the patient tell you as much as she wants to share, and they open the door for her to speak seriously of her inner feelings if she is comfortable doing so.

If you know the person well and want to offer spiritual comfort, bookstores have a number of books that are appropriate as gifts. The patient can read the book when she feels up to it and is ready for the message. During the first year after my diagnosis with multiple sclerosis, I received three copies of *When Bad Things Happen to Good People*. I was ready to read it in the second year; it's a great book.

Check with your bookstore, minister, or other spiritual counselor, or with the patient's family, for appropriate inspirational gift ideas.

Seeing the Person, Not the Illness

From the patient's perspective, one of the hardest things to handle after being diagnosed with a disease is the tendency for people to see you as your disease, not the multifaceted person you are. Yes, you do have a disease, but you also have a family, a job, hobbies, a home, and interests far beyond any physical limitations.

Fourteen years after my diagnosis with multiple sclerosis, there are still people who can only talk to me about MS or make comments about how good I look. I work hard to look good so that people will see beyond my illness, and most people with chronic diseases do the same. With the exception of people who have some notable mind-robbers like Alzheimer's disease, most people with chronic diseases have all their mental faculties. Yet some people talk about the patient in the third person, even when she is present. This is especially true if obvious physical symptoms are present. It is as if the person has become invisible or is unable to speak for herself: "Would she like more coffee?" "How is she feeling?" "Has this been a hard winter for her?"

Wheelchair users face similar problems. They are often treated as if their minds went when they lost the use of their legs. They are addressed in baby talk or called "dear." Very often people raise their voices when talking to a chair user, as if she is hard of hearing. She may have trouble walking, but most chair users can hear just fine.

Thoughtlessness is not limited to the patients themselves. About nine months after Nicholas was diagnosed, a friend saw Buffy for the first time, and blurted out, "You're looking well." How was she supposed to look?

There are cases when an illness, such as Alzheimer's and similar diseases, does affect the patient's mind. In this case "It's nice to see you" is a good way to open a conversation. This patient struggles to respond to questions, and it is most thoughtful to present subjects without forming a question she has to answer. Your statement allows her to respond or not, as her condition permits that day.

The important thing is to treat each person as an individual and to relate to her as she is at the moment. Be thoughtful of her condition and of her real limitations, but guard against judging her based on stereotypes.

Follow the Rules

In addition to visiting hours, the hospital may place other restrictions on visitors, for the good of the patient.

Intensive care units limit the amount of time people can visit, often to five or ten minutes an hour. Stick to it. Don't expect the hospital personnel to be your time clock; they have more important work to do. As an adult you should take responsibility for yourself.

When my mother was in a coronary care unit I became so frustrated by her friends, who would not leave until the nurse came in and kicked them out. It is rude to stay beyond your allotted time, and this often can set back the patient's recovery.

In some cases the patient will ask or even beg you to stay. Before agreeing, check with the nurse on duty. The patient may want company, but that may not be what is best for her. Let the patient know that you are nearby and will be in again during the next visiting hour.

Another visiting requirement may be to wear masks, usually paper masks with elastic to hook them over the ears. They can be uncomfortable, but are required when the patient is susceptible to infection and needs protection from germs you may not even know you have. One man who called on Nicholas felt fine the day of his visit, but the next day came down with a bad case of stomach flu. Fortunately, he had worn a mask during his visit, and Nick avoided a major setback.

Mary's mother shared a compelling story with me. Mary was in isolation with a 104° temperature, an extremely low blood count, and an immune system that had virtually shut down. She was allowed visits only from parents and grandparents, and even they were required to wear a gown, mask, and hat to enter the room. Visitors who left the room had to put on all new covering before reentering. "Mary's grandmother came to the hospital to see her but didn't want to bother putting on 'all that stuff' so she stood outside the room and waved to Mary through the window." The first time Grandma did this, Mary's mother left the sickroom, took off all her "equipment," and visited with Grandma. After that, mother decided she would not leave Mary alone just because Grandma was unwilling to do as small a thing as putting on protective covering. "From that point on I stayed with Mary and let Grandma stand outside and wave at us. I told Mary I felt like a monkey in the zoo, and that was the first smile I had seen in weeks."

Visiting at Home

Many of the suggestions discussed for hospital visits apply to home visits as well, except that there are no visiting hours to control the time you stay. If you don't police your own visit, you may stay longer than is good for the patient.

Call ahead before you visit to ensure that you are coming at a convenient time. Your call also alerts the patient to clean up, because company's coming. I often wear a robe over my nightgown if I don't feel well and don't expect anyone to visit. Sometimes I look a little ragged. I appreciate the opportunity get presentable before guests arrive.

Normally, if the patient is feeling better, you can stay longer and participate in activities to entertain the patient. The patient's condition and energy level should always dictate the length of the visit. When she starts to fade, it's time to leave.

Always remember that you are there for the patient. We asked earlier "Why are you there?" with regard to hospital visits. The same question must be raised regarding home visits. We have heard stories of people bringing a six-pack of beer and settling in for the evening, staying long past the patient's bedtime. If you are seeking entertainment, go to a movie.

In Closing

Visiting a patient can be one of the most important things you do. You will brighten her day and help the time pass, but be sure you always keep in mind her best interests.

What Can You Do to Help?

✓ Visit only if you are comfortable doing so. If you are afraid of hospitals or get sick from the smells, stay home. The patient has better things to do than worry about you.

✓ Be prepared with conversation ideas so you can keep things light and interesting, without expecting the patient to contribute more than she is able. If she feels like talking, you can save your conversation ideas for another time.

✓ Follow visiting hours, special intensive care hours, and any other rules that may be established for the good of the patient. Wear masks and other protective clothing when it is required.

✓ Do not offer false hope or tell a patient she'll be just fine when you know she is dying. Do not speak in trite phrases or tell the patient how she should feel. Ask open-ended questions that allow the patient to tell you how she is feeling and where she finds her strength.

✓ Keep the person in the forefront of your thinking. Do not diminish her as a person by considering her only in terms of her illness.

Chapter Ten

When Reaching Out Is Difficult

Illness and disease raise many issues for us. We may be afraid, turned off, or uncomfortable around people with certain illnesses. Unable to see the total person, we may become so obsessed with the illness that it is the only thing we relate to.

A lot of our ideas about illness are rooted in ignorance. Medical advances have cleared up many mysteries about certain illnesses, yet our personal knowledge base may not have kept up. If our information is based on 1950s data, we may be drawing conclusions that are totally inappropriate based on the information available today.

When someone close to you becomes ill, it is important to have the best and most current information. Learn as much as you can about the illness to address any fears you may have and also to be of the most help to the patient. The more you know, the better able you will be to provide understanding and practical assistance.

Fear of Illness

Some illnesses or disabilities may frighten us, and we may turn away from a friend if he is diagnosed with that disease. I had a dear friend who lived in another community but with whom I had stayed in regular contact. I never heard from her again after I told her I had MS.

Cancer patients often relate a similar story. Friends are afraid they will catch it, are frightened by the prospect of a terminal illness, or are afraid of the unknown. Whatever the fear, the result is that a friend is deprived of the companionship he needs at a critical time in his life.

Sam was so uncomfortable with the idea of cancer that he never visited a lifelong friend, Will, who was dying of the disease. Will could not understand Sam or figure out what was wrong. It was a source of great sadness to him at a time when he was experiencing enough sadness.

This situation is a tragedy for all involved. The patient is deprived of friendship and support from those he needs most. He feels betrayed and alone, and is afraid others will leave him as well. He may stop telling people about his illness, or may put on a happy face so he will not lose any other friends. The person who carries the fear and turns away from his friend feels guilt, remorse, and great sorrow at the situation. His respect for himself is diminished.

Illnesses with a Stigma

Some illnesses, like AIDS, carry a stigma. Because the disease is sometimes transmitted through activity that society might not condone, a person may lack compassion for all people who are battling its effects. By blaming the victim he loses sight of the suffering the patient is experiencing and may turn his back on a friend who needs his help.

Many of us engage in activities that jeopardize our health: smoking, drinking to excess, and obesity, to name a few. Yet we do not turn away from a lung cancer patient simply because he was a smoker, or reject an obese person when he develops heart trouble. We may wish he had not engaged in harmful behaviors, but that doesn't stop us from helping him now.

A part of our reluctance to help may also come from not know-ing if there are special ways to treat a person with AIDS, or similar diseases. In chapter 6 ideas for helping a person with a chronic or ter-minal illness are discussed. These ideas are appropriate regardless of the nature of the illness.

Mental illness is another situation in which stigma often gets in the way of support. People who have an emotional illness need every bit as much support as those who have a physical illness, yet once again the fear of the disease may prevent friends from offering sup-port. In this case, the fear often comes from a lack of understanding about the illness and its causes. Try to learn more about the illness. You will likely find that your level of comfort will increase.

Sound helping principles apply regardless of the nature of the ill-ness. If you would send flowers to a patient in a medical hospital, send the same to a friend in a mental hospital. If a patient is depressed, reaching out by phone, card, or visit will likely be appre-ciated as well.

Overcoming Fear or Stigma

When you are faced with someone who has an illness you find emo-tionally difficult to handle, there are ways you can work to overcome your resistance. Educate yourself about the disease. How is it trans-mitted? Are you at risk? Are there precautions you can take if it is contagious? Many local, state, and national organizations exist to help patients with specific diseases to educate their families and friends. You can find these groups in your community by looking in the Yellow Pages. Call or visit the office to find out what information is available; talk with the staff. The more you know, the less frightening the illness will be. Your family doctor is another good source for information specific to your risk.

Talk with family or friends of other people who have the disease. Talk with your sick friend's family. Talk with the patient himself; ask him what he is experiencing.

Your minister, priest, or rabbi may be helpful, particularly if you see the illness as a moral issue. He can put the illness in a religious perspective and can tell you what your faith believes about the disease. A mental health professional or other counselor can discuss your fears with you and can help you find their origins. Many times our fears are rooted in things we were told as children or the language used at the time. Mentally ill people were called "mad"; people confined to wheelchairs or otherwise disabled were call "invalid." Thankfully, many things have changed for the better in recent years, including our language.

Whatever the nature of the illness, people are hurting and need all the support and help they can get. If the patient is a friend or family member, and we truly want to help, it is important to overcome our fears and biases, to recognize that the person who is ill today is the same person we knew and loved yesterday. That person has not changed.

If you are uncomfortable or afraid, don't cut the patient off completely. Send a card now and then, or send a basket of flowers. It will let him know he is in your thoughts. Call if you can. You don't have to take an active role in his recovery to stay in touch. It may be that after you have communicated for a while through mail and phone, you will feel more comfortable about visiting.

In Closing

Sometimes a friend's illness strikes at our own fears, prejudices, and ignorance. We may be uncomfortable with the illness and therefore be unable to relate to the patient at a human level.

What Can You Do to Help?

- ✓ Make sure you have current information about the disease. Ask doctors, family, and the patient for background, or contact organizations that support people with that disease.
- ✓ Realize that the person is hurting and needs your help. Don't turn your back on the patient because you don't like his disease.
- ✓ Treat the patient with respect, and follow the same helping guidelines you would use in helping a person with any illness.

Chapter Eleven

Special Situations—
Innovative Solutions

In a book of this kind it is difficult to cover every circumstance that might arise for a patient or her family. Some situations require such innovative solutions that a separate chapter seemed in order.

Financial Needs

Illness can create a terrible financial burden. If you have a friend who is struggling financially, giving money may be the most appropriate thing you can do. If you can help financially, you may be a lifesaver. In order to donate or spend the money most appropriately, it is wise to seek direction from a person close to the situation.

When the patient has limited health insurance, or needs a treatment that is considered experimental and is not covered by insurance, it may be necessary to raise large sums of money to cover current bills and to provide for the future. Concerned friends often find innovative ways to help. People have organized bake sales, car washes, garage sales, golf tournaments, bingo nights, and fund-raising breakfasts or dinners.

When fund-raising efforts are needed, start by considering what your community enjoys doing or what activities have been most successful as fund-raisers in the past. These options might include bowling, golf, tennis, walking, running, a read-a-thon, bridge tournament, bingo, or a similar activity. Try to select the kind of event that people enjoy, but one that is not overused. If your town already has a series of runs for special causes, think of something different: a special performance of a play or showing of a movie, a bowling tournament, or a concert by a favorite group. There are as many ideas as people to think of them, and you'll be surprised at the number of people who are willing to help.

Other community resources can be contacted to help. Businesses often will underwrite the expenses for fund-raising events in return for a mention in promotional materials. Firms are even more likely to help if they have a connection with the family. Churches and service organizations may have special funds to assist as well. Find out if the patient's family members belong to any associations that could be contacted for support.

Another source of support may be local radio or television personalities, who are often willing to lend their names to charitable events. They may also be willing to mention your fund-raising event on their programs.

Local newspapers, radio, and television stations often run community calendars that list upcoming events. They should be notified of your event so it can be included. You may be able to interest a local reporter in your event, and she may be willing to do stories both before and after the event.

It will be important to have a committee that actually runs the event and shares the workload. Goodwill stretches thin when there are not enough volunteers to do the work. You will also need one person to serve as chair to keep the project on track and to arbitrate disputes.

Fund-raising is an activity in which everyone—regardless of

age—can participate. While adults may be working on a dinner with a large ticket price, young people can organize a car wash or similar fund-raising effort. Classmates, church groups, and youth organizations should be offered the opportunity to get involved. It will be a wonderful learning experience as well as a fun activity.

One young man in our community was hit by lightning on a golf course. He was not expected to live because the damage to his system was so severe. He did survive and is very alert, though he requires around-the-clock care. His parents have put their careers on hold to care for him, and an annual celebrity golf tournament raises enough money each year to allow them to provide the care he needs and to support the family. Many community leaders and area celebrities come together to assure the event's success.

A Team Approach

A friend was driving home from work on a cold, icy evening. As she approached a familiar curve in the road, a dog walked into the middle of the street. She slammed on her brakes, skidded, turned over in a ditch. When she woke up several days later, she no longer had the use of her legs.

This catastrophic situation required a team of people—medical professionals, family, friends, and the community—to help the patient put her life back together. The house had to be redesigned, the car was replaced with a van specially equipped with hand controls, and the patient had to learn to care for herself and to create a new life with more limitations than she ever imagined.

When a crisis of this kind strikes, pull together friends who are willing to serve as a support system and to help with all the tasks that must be accomplished. Make a list of the jobs that need to be done, then assign each member of the team responsibility for gathering information on one or two of the areas listed. In the case given above, assignments might include investigating the best rehabilitation facilities in the area; contacting companies that make vans with hand controls and determining the costs involved; finding driving classes to teach the patient to use the van; looking for architects to develop the plans for modifying the house to be wheelchair accessible; locating a support group for persons with her kind of disability; identifying community groups that offer specific assistance she needs; and so on.

The team will also be the patient's support system, visiting regularly, calling, and sending cards. A list of members' phone numbers should be given to the patient so she has people to call when she is lonely or needs help or companionship.

The team approach to a potentially terminal illness was discussed in chapter 6. The idea of a team is appropriate whenever a major crisis occurs. Instead of a small group of friends helping out, the broader resources of the community can be brought together. That way duplication is avoided, and the best information available can be brought to each situation. The support team can be critical to the patient's full recovery. With them all things are possible; without them, the patient often has a bleak future.

An Illness Out of Town

An illness or accident can strike anyplace, at any time. When a friend is many miles away, there may be little you can do directly, but ways you can help from afar.

If you have a friend in the area, call and ask her to check on your friend. Seeing a friendly face, even one you don't know, can be reassuring when you are in a strange community. If the patient is active in a church, call that denomination in the town where she is ill. It is likely that the rector or a lay leader will be glad to pay a call. Send flowers, cards, and other reminders that you are thinking of her.

It may be that the best way to help the patient is to help her family. They may be traveling to care for her and will need help getting ready to leave, help with errands or household tasks, a ride to the airport, or assistance in looking after the house while they are gone. For a comprehensive list of ideas for helping the family, see chapter 8.

When one man was hospitalized 350 miles from home, a friend offered to fly there and drive him home in his own car. The offer was most thoughtful, as the patient was weak after his illness and would have had difficulty getting home on his own.

In Closing

Not all illnesses are alike, and at times the help that is needed requires innovation and the combined resources of many people and organizations.

What Can You Do to Help?

✓ Work together to raise money when it is needed. Involve family, friends, community leaders, businesses, and young people in fund-raising efforts.

✓ Use a team approach by bringing all the resources of the community together to help a person with a catastrophic illness or injury.

✓ In each situation look for what is needed; then take a creative approach to meeting those needs.

Closing Thoughts

No magic formula exists that will help you help others. In each case it is a matter of people reaching out in the best way they know how, one person to another.

If this book has one message, it is: Just do it. Do what you can, when you can, based on your personal circumstances at the time. In one case you may only be able to send a card; in another you may make a meal. The next time you can stay with the patient while the caregiver has lunch. The important thing is to recognize a need and to meet it.

You can't do the wrong thing. Every genuine act will be appreciated because you did it. The patient and the family are grateful for the kind acts of others that make their lives a little easier and brighter.

What Can You Do to Help?

✓ In every illness situation there will be ways to help; you only have to look for them.

✓ Consider the age and circumstances of the person you want to help.

✓ Consider your personal resources. How much time do you have to help, and what are you in a position to contribute? Can you clean the house, mow the lawn, write a card, walk the dog, visit the hospital, or play a game with the patient?

✓ Don't offer to do more than you are able to do. If you only have time to send a card, that's fine. It will be appreciated.

✓ If you are unsure what needs to be done, ask. A family member or a close friend can often provide ideas for things that are needed. Look around; often the things we need to do around our own home are things a patient or family needs done as well.

✓ Stay in touch with a card, call, or visit.

✓ Don't forget the patient who has an illness that continues for an extended period of time, or who is in a nursing home. Make sure the patient is included in family decisions and is made to feel a part of the larger community. Write yourself notes to remember.

✓ Remember brothers and sisters of children who are ill, and remember the caregivers. They make sacrifices that often go unnoticed, and they will appreciate having their contribution recognized.